Welcome

If you've been told you need to monitor your blood pressure, or if it's something you want to take control of before it becomes an issue, you've picked up the right book. With so much information out there, it can feel overwhelming, which is why we've put together a comprehensive guide where everything you need to know is all in one place. From understanding the science behind hypertension and what actually happens to your body, to exploring the causes, risk factors and implications of having high blood pressure, we've got it all covered. Discover how to make small changes to your lifestyle that will have a big impact on your health, and check out ten simple and delicious recipes, which are perfect for managing your blood pressure. So, delve in and start to take back control of your health today.

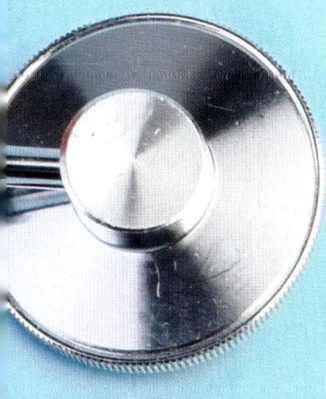

CONTENTS

06
GET TO GRIPS WITH HYPERTENSION

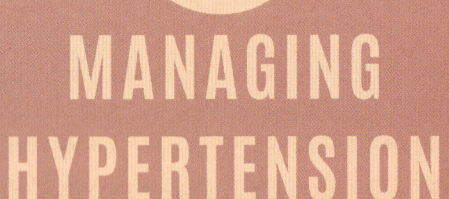

1 UNDERSTANDING HYPERTENSION

10
BLOOD PRESSURE EXPLAINED

16
MYTHBUSTING HYPERTENSION

18
WHAT ABOUT CHOLESTEROL?

20
CAUSES AND RISK FACTORS

26
SECONDARY HYPERTENSION

30
RISKS AND HEALTH IMPLICATIONS

36
GETTING A DIAGNOSIS

40
SIGNS AND SYMPTOMS

2 MANAGING HYPERTENSION

48
YOUR TREATMENT OPTIONS

52
MEDICATIONS FOR HYPERTENSION

56
WEIGHT MANAGEMENT

62
STRESS AND HYPERTENSION

66
MANAGING ALCOHOL CONSUMPTION

70
SMOKING AND HYPERTENSION

74
SUPPORT GROUPS AND RESOURCES

3 LIFESTYLE

78 OPTIMISE YOUR LIFESTYLE

82 THE IMPORTANCE OF PHYSICAL ACTIVITY

88 THE BEST TYPES OF EXERCISE FOR HYPERTENSION

92 IMPROVE YOUR SLEEP

96 HOW TO EAT FOR HYPERTENSION

102 TOP 10 FOODS FOR HYPERTENSION

4 RECIPES

110 CHOCOLATE AND HAZELNUT GRANOLA

112 SUPER BERRY BREAKFAST BOWL

114 SPICED CARROT AND LENTIL SOUP

116 TUNA AND LENTIL SALAD

118 SPICY BEEF AND LENTIL CHILLI

120 CHICKEN AND KALE STIR-FRY

122 SICILIAN-STYLE MACKEREL

124 OAT-AND-SESAME-CRUSTED SALMON WITH BLISTERED TOMATOES

126 VEGGIE CURRY WITH A MINTY YOGHURT

128 NUT, SEED AND BERRY CRUMBLE

INTRODUCTION

GET TO GRIPS WITH HYPERTENSION

Your in-depth guide to understanding, managing and controlling your blood pressure starts here

If you've picked up this title, then chances are you're worried about high blood pressure. That might be because you have recently been diagnosed yourself, you've been warned that you're in a pre-hypertension state (ie at risk of having high blood pressure), or you have someone close to you with hypertension. There's a lot of different information out there about high blood pressure and it can be overwhelming trying to plough through it all and figure out what you need to do and where to start. That's why we've done the hard work for you; scouring the latest advice and research, and pulling it together into one handbook.

'Knowledge is power', as the saying goes. The more you know about what your blood pressure is, what it means when it's too high, and how we read blood pressure, the better you'll be able to understand the condition and start to think about how to get it under control. Quite often, the literature we are given from a doctor upon diagnosis focuses only on how to treat a condition and the risks, rather than what's happening within our bodies. It's also important to know what can happen if blood pressure is left untreated – but it's not intended to scare you; just to make you aware of the possible complications. Being able to know and spot the signs of anything serious means you're able to alert someone and get medical help far more quickly.

There are two main pathways for treating high blood pressure once it's been diagnosed: lifestyle changes and medication. You may already be on medication for hypertension or had a conversation with your doctor about it, and we have a section explaining the key types of treatment and how they work so you can understand what they are doing. Whether you're on medication or not, you're probably also looking at making some changes within your life to help reduce your blood pressure further and bring it under control. That's why we have dedicated a whole section to improving your lifestyle, covering everything from food and exercise, to sleep and stress. As diet can play such a big role in managing blood pressure, we've also selected some great recipes that will nourish your body, support your health and give you fresh inspiration.

The benefits of this go far beyond managing your blood pressure. A healthy lifestyle also helps to reduce your risk of things like type 2 diabetes, heart problems, stroke, dementia, mental health conditions, some cancers and stress. When you work with your body and give it what it needs, you will find that you have more energy, better focus and improved sleep. And the best bit is that even the smallest of changes can have a huge impact, and making lots of little changes in different areas will all combine to have a cumulative effect on your overall health.

Just remember that you're in control, so while we've tried to include everything in this book, you can pick and choose which sections are most relevant to you to build your own personal hypertension plan.

YOUR JOURNEY
Do what's right for you to manage your blood pressure; everyone will tackle their health differently.

GET TO GRIPS WITH HYPERTENSION

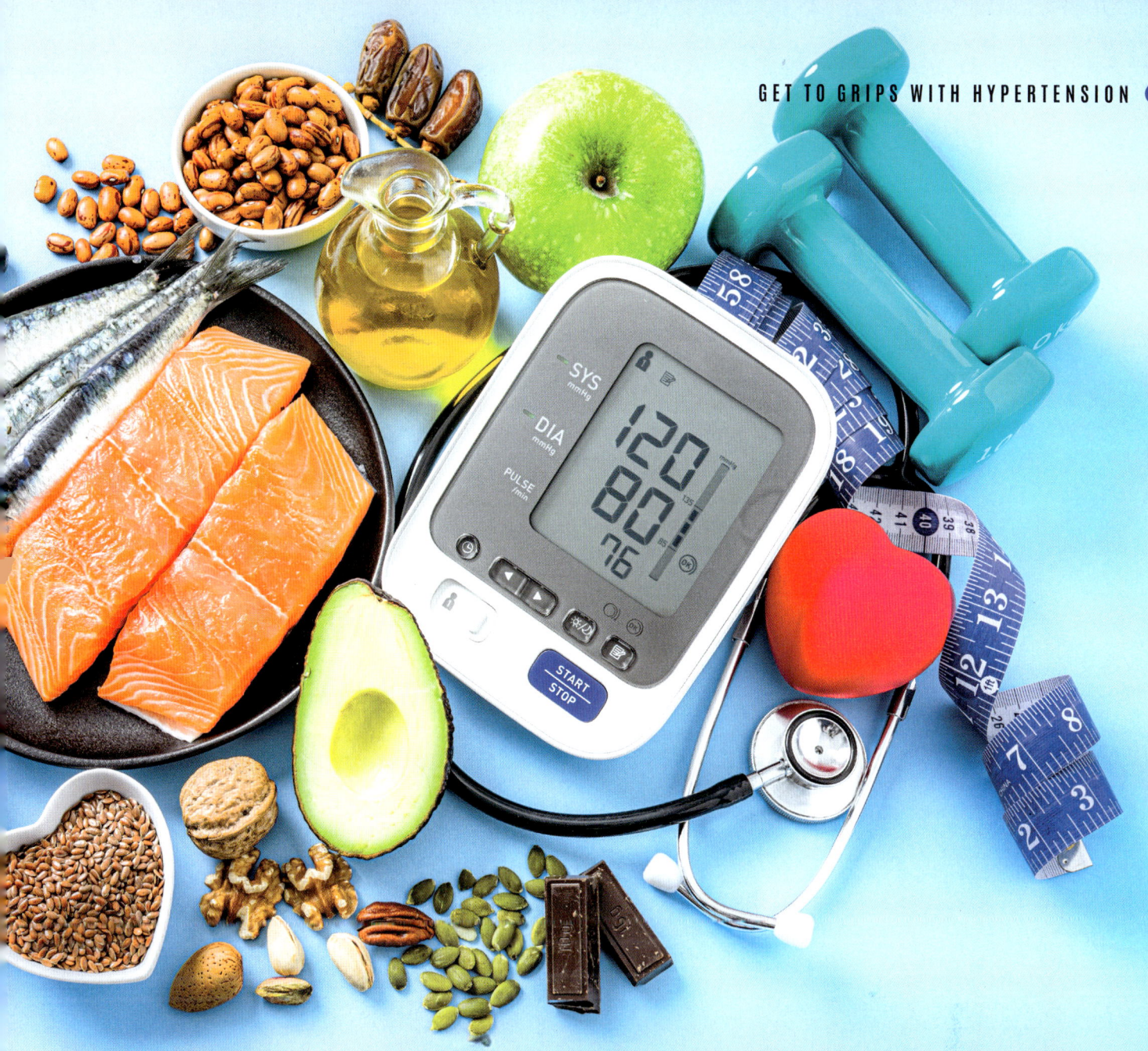

PROOF THAT INTERVENTION WORKS!

Research demonstrates that making lifestyle modifications is effective for improving hypertension

It can be scary to find out you have high blood pressure, especially when the news headlines focus on things like heart attack and stroke as a consequence of hypertension. But it's not too late to make changes, and there is plenty of data to support the fact that you can improve your blood pressure readings with lifestyle changes. One research article[1] looked in detail at how effective the guidelines for dealing with hypertension are. In short, these guidelines include doing regular exercise, reducing your intake of salt, alcohol and smoking, and eating a healthy diet – specifically the DASH diet, which is a nutrition plan developed for hypertensive patients (don't worry, we cover this in more detail). The article states that one of the trials it reviewed found that: 'The DASH diet, combined with alcohol and salt reduction, weight loss, and aerobic exercise, achieved a reduction of 14.2/7.4 mmHg among hypertensives, while hypertension prevalence fell over a period of 6 months from 38% to 12%'. That's a significant statistic and means that any changes you make will be hugely worthwhile.

[1] Hypertension and Lifestyle Modification: How Useful are the Guidelines? Br J Gen Pract. December 2010

UNDERSTANDING HYPERTENSION

Discover the science behind blood pressure, what it means and why it should be taken seriously

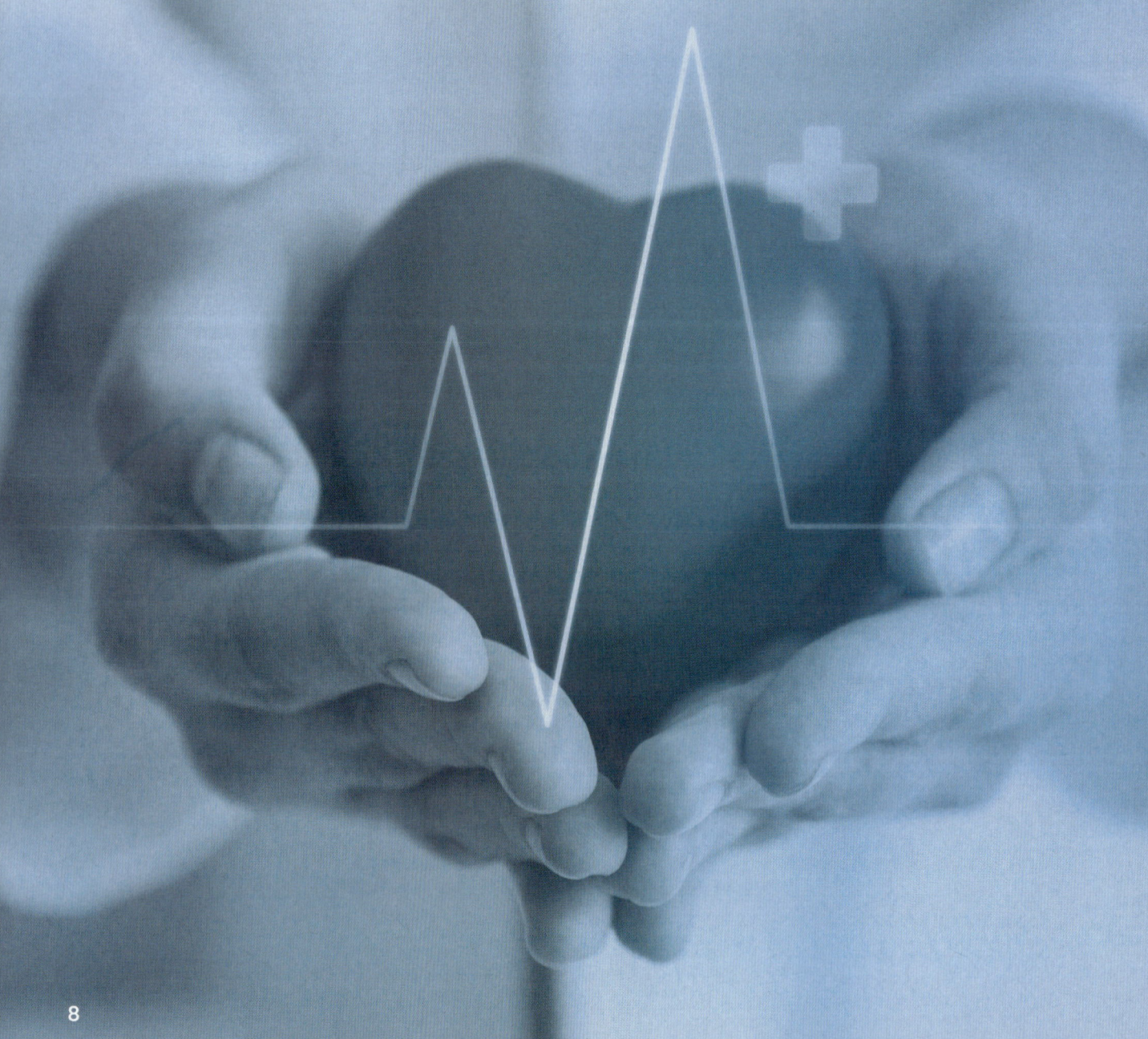

1

10
BLOOD PRESSURE EXPLAINED

16
MYTHBUSTING HYPERTENSION

18
WHAT ABOUT CHOLESTEROL?

20
CAUSES AND RISK FACTORS

26
SECONDARY HYPERTENSION

30
RISKS AND HEALTH IMPLICATIONS

36
GETTING A DIAGNOSIS

40
SIGNS AND SYMPTOMS

UNDERSTANDING
HYPERTENSION

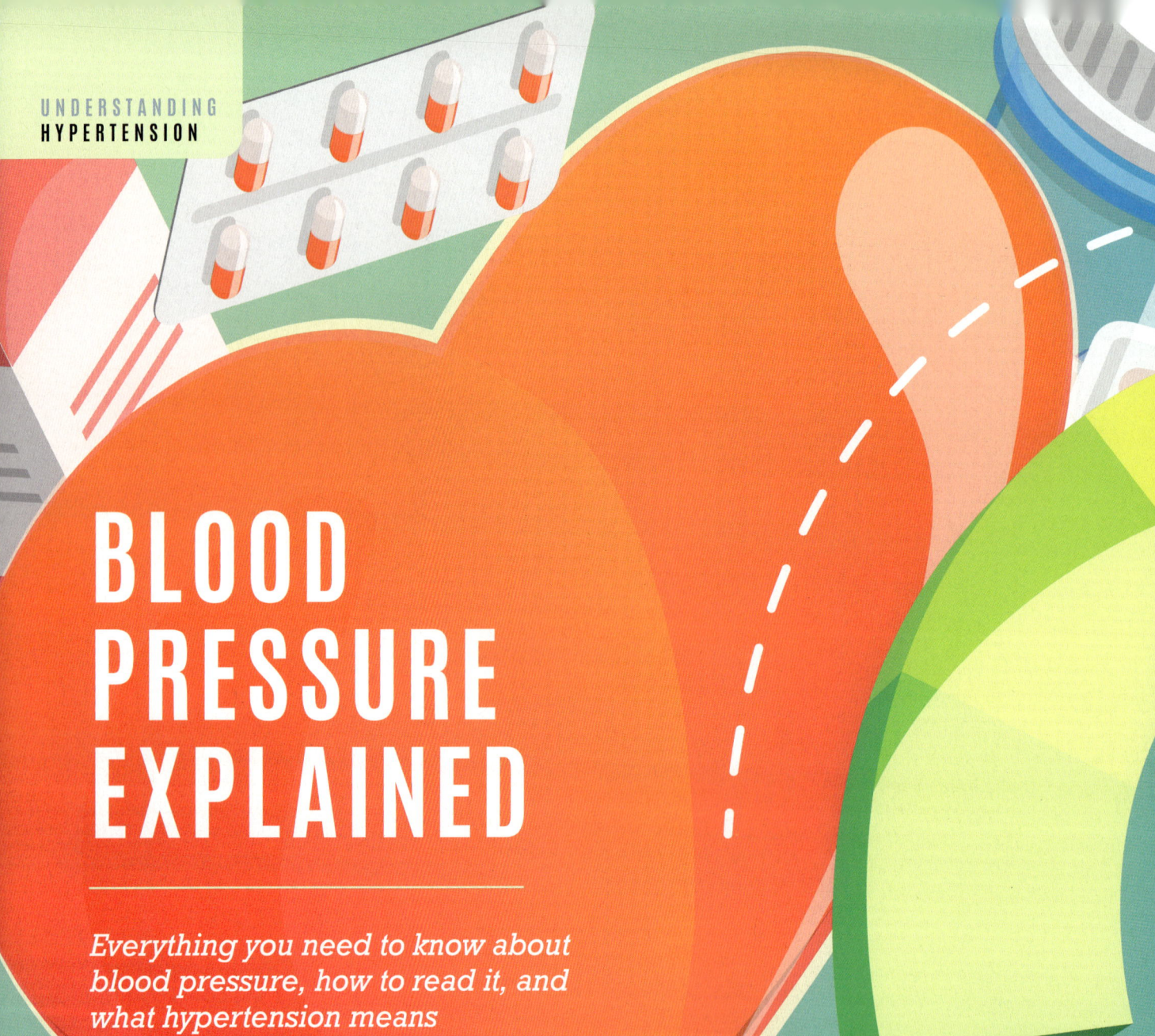

BLOOD PRESSURE EXPLAINED

Everything you need to know about blood pressure, how to read it, and what hypertension means

When it comes to monitoring your health, there are various useful metrics that you should keep an eye on. One of the most important is your blood pressure, as this can indicate the state of your overall health in addition to your potential risk of future health complications. It's something that is easy, quick and free to check, but can tell you a lot about your wellbeing.

Blood pressure is exactly what it sounds like: it's the pressure of your blood in your arteries. A quick biology lesson – arteries are blood vessels, consisting of tube-like structures that carry blood away from the heart, transporting oxygen and nutrients around your body and to the brain. Blood is then transported back to the heart through your veins once the oxygen has been depleted. Your heart is responsible for pumping this blood around your body, and it's important to maintain good blood pressure to ensure all your body's systems are working optimally. Arteries can stretch to accommodate changes in your blood pressure; problems occur when your arteries become stiff or narrow, preventing them from being as flexible.

Blood pressure will change throughout the day and night; it's not fixed. Things like eating and drinking, physical activity, stress and anxiety, or even whether you're standing or sitting, can have a short-term impact on your blood pressure. Blood pressure also naturally increases with age, as blood vessels begin to thicken and

10

BLOOD PRESSURE EXPLAINED

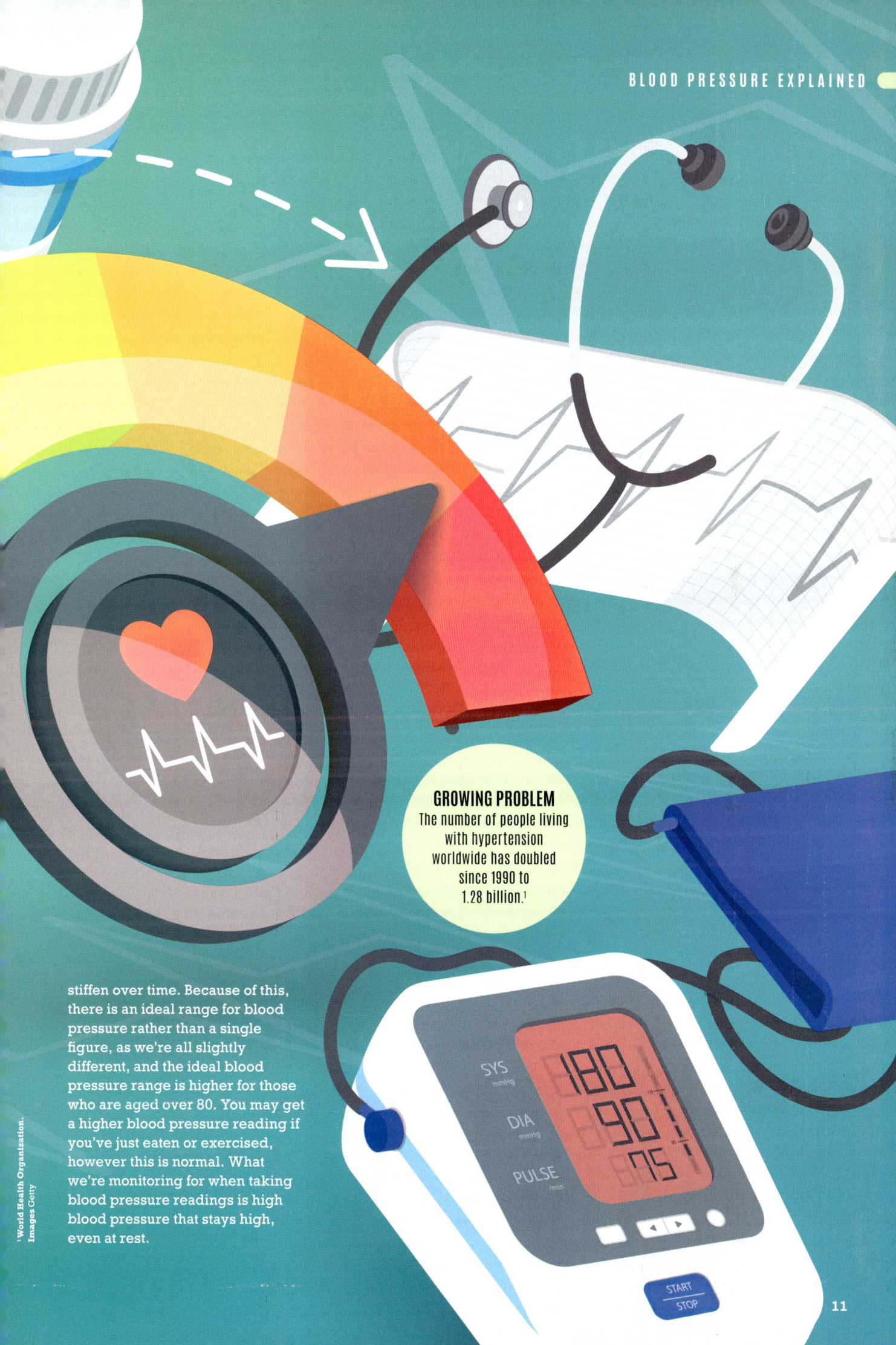

GROWING PROBLEM
The number of people living with hypertension worldwide has doubled since 1990 to 1.28 billion.[1]

stiffen over time. Because of this, there is an ideal range for blood pressure rather than a single figure, as we're all slightly different, and the ideal blood pressure range is higher for those who are aged over 80. You may get a higher blood pressure reading if you've just eaten or exercised, however this is normal. What we're monitoring for when taking blood pressure readings is high blood pressure that stays high, even at rest.

[1] World Health Organization. Images Getty

UNDERSTANDING
HYPERTENSION

BUYING ADVICE FOR BLOOD PRESSURE MACHINES

Know what to look for in an at-home monitor

Given how important monitoring your blood pressure is, you might be considering purchasing your own blood pressure machine so you can keep an eye on your readings more frequently. Home machines are undoubtably very convenient, but before you rush out and buy one, it's worth bearing in mind that you need to be sure you're doing it correctly to get accurate results, so read the instructions or ask a professional to show you how to use it. You also need to be aware that different machines have different features. The most basic ones, and therefore the cheapest, will have a cuff to put on your arm, linked to a simple monitor screen to display your readings. You can also buy machines that use wrist cuffs, but unless you have a reason why you can't use an upper arm cuff, this is the best type to use. You must also check the cuff size to ensure that it fits snugly around your arm; you can measure your arm with a tape measure to help when shopping for monitors online. Also check that the monitor you have chosen is approved in your country – for example, in the UK, you are looking for one that has been validated as accurate by the British and Irish Hypertension Society (BIHS). On more expensive monitors, your readings may be recorded digitally, or synced with an app or computer, but you can keep a written record.

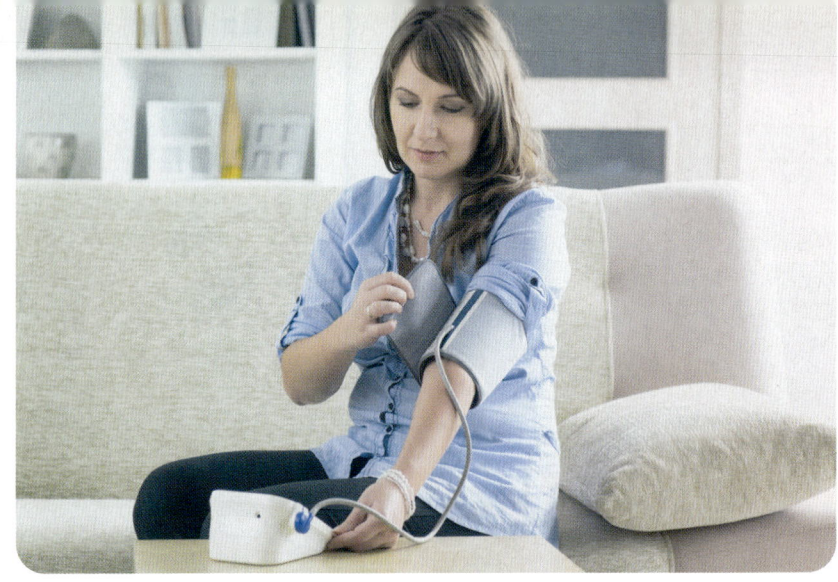

MEASURING BLOOD PRESSURE

Because blood pressure is such an important measure of health, it's something that we all should be aware of and keeping an eye on regularly. High blood pressure can happen to anyone, though there are certain risk factors (which we'll cover in more detail later in this book), but it becomes more common with age. However, many people have never been checked and have no idea what their blood pressure is. The only way to know if your blood pressure is in the normal range, is to have a blood pressure check.

For those under 40, it's a good idea to do this to give you an idea of your health. This also gives a good starting number to monitor any changes. From the age of 40, it's wise to have a blood pressure check at least every five years if you're otherwise healthy and have a normal blood pressure reading. If your blood pressure readings start to creep up, or you're at the higher end of the normal range, then it's better to get your blood pressure checked every year. Those who have been diagnosed with high blood pressure may have far more frequent checks.

It's very simple and painless to have your blood pressure checked. It usually involves having a cuff secured around your upper arm. This is then inflated until it's tight, which can be a little uncomfortable for a few seconds, and then the blood pressure reading can be taken. Sometimes this is taken manually by a clinical professional using a stethoscope to listen to your blood pressure, but more often it will be an automatic device with a screen to show the readings. It's a very quick process, but it's important to be relaxed and to not talk while the blood pressure is being recorded.

When your blood pressure has been read, there will be two numbers. The first of these is called systolic pressure, which is the higher number, and this is the pressure against your arteries as your heart pumps blood through them. The second is the diastolic pressure, the lower number, which is the pressure in your arteries between heart beats, ie when it's relaxed and not pumping blood. Your readings will be given as '[systolic] over [diastolic]'. The higher your numbers, the harder the heart is having to work to pump blood around the body. There is a normal range for these numbers, which means that your heart is working optimally, and this is good for your overall health and wellbeing. If you're not within this normal range, then this is something that does need to be addressed – sometimes urgently.

BLOOD PRESSURE EXPLAINED

HIGH BLOOD PRESSURE

The main reason we measure blood pressure is to look for high readings. High blood pressure can be a very serious condition, and it can have no symptoms. Many people with high blood pressure are unaware of it. If your arteries stiffen, this can make it easier for fatty deposits to build up, and this can lead to serious health complications including heart attack, stroke, kidney failure or vascular dementia. In fact, according to the British Heart Foundation, 50% of heart attacks and strokes are associated with high blood pressure.

This all sounds scary, but it is why we should carry out regular checks. We can often see the danger signs of rising blood pressure and can make the necessary lifestyle changes or treatment plans to prevent it from getting any worse.

High blood pressure is also called hypertension, and there are different stages. In the box on page 15 we have a useful chart that shows you what these different stages look like and how to plot your own readings, but here we'll explain the stages in more detail.

Normal blood pressure

This is considered as readings between 90/60 mmHG and 120/80 mmHG. However, for those aged over 80, it's not unusual to be higher than this, so ideal is considered as readings under 150/90 mmHG. If you're in this range, then this indicates that blood pressure is optimal and is a good sign for future health outcomes. However, chances are that if you've picked up this book then you're not within this range right now, but it's good to know what numbers you're aiming for.

Pre-hypertension

This refers to readings that are slightly too high, but not quite in the high blood pressure range. This is for readings between 120/80 mmHG and 140/90 mmHG, and can act as a warning sign to start taking measures to prevent it from getting any higher and becoming a problem.

Stage 1 hypertension

This is the first level of high blood pressure, with a reading of between 140/90 mmHG and 160/100 mmHG. At this stage, you might not need to take any medication or other treatments, but you should start taking active steps towards lifestyle changes to bring these numbers down. Bear in mind that the threshold for blood pressure readings is lower if you're taking them yourself at home to allow for inaccuracies, so in this case the range for Stage 1 would be 135/85 mmHG and 150/95 mmHG.

Stage 2 hypertension

You enter the stage 2 range when your readings are between 160/100 mmHG and 180/120 mmHG (or over 150/95 mmHG if taking the reading at home). This requires intervention to ensure that it doesn't go any higher and to start to lower those numbers towards a healthier range.

Stage 3 hypertension

This is also called 'severe hypertension' and refers to a systolic pressure reading over 180 mmHG or a diastolic reading over 120 mmHG taken in a clinical setting. This is considered a serious condition and needs urgent referral for investigation and treatment.

It's unusual to be diagnosed with high blood pressure based on a single reading, as readings can fluctuate throughout a day. We cover this more in our section on diagnosis later on.

While this book looks at high blood pressure, to give full context, we also want to mention low blood pressure. Low blood pressure is when you have a reading of less than 90/60 mmHG. This is also called hypotension and can lead to symptoms like feeling dizzy, getting lightheaded, feeling sick, blurred vision, fainting or feeling weak. This can be caused by things like certain medications, some medical conditions or pregnancy (which can also be a cause of high blood pressure).

13

UNDERSTANDING
HYPERTENSION

WORRY OVER HIGH BLOOD PRESSURE

If you're diagnosed with high blood pressure, then it's only natural to feel a little worried, especially when it comes to considering the possible health risks and complications. We will talk more about causes and risk factors elsewhere in this book, but regardless of the reasons behind your high blood pressure, it's important to know that you can do something about it and improve your health.

Even fit and healthy people can be diagnosed with high blood pressure; it's a very common condition. There are some risk factors, such as age, race and genetics, that you can do nothing about. However, many of the risk factors that contribute towards high blood pressure are things that you can take control of. You have the power to bring your blood pressure down and reduce your risk of future health complications. If you're working with a healthcare team, it can be a good idea to set goals around what you want to achieve, such as a target blood pressure reading to aim for. This can help when it comes to staying motivated.

It can also help to put into place a plan of action, setting out goals in key areas. For example, you might set fitness goals, nutrition goals and activity goals, which will all contribute to your overall success. And by making these kinds of lifestyle changes, it can also help improve your health in other areas.

You may also find it useful to keep a diary of your blood pressure readings. This can help you to learn any patterns, such as whether you get higher readings at certain times of the day or after doing certain things. Keeping track also helps you to see improvements visually, which can keep you working towards your ultimate goal. You may also benefit from seeking support, by talking to someone you trust or to your healthcare team – we talk more about support groups and resources later on.

Hopefully you now have a better understanding of high blood pressure, what it means and how it's measured. The more you know, the better prepared you can be, and the more likely you are to succeed in controlling your health.

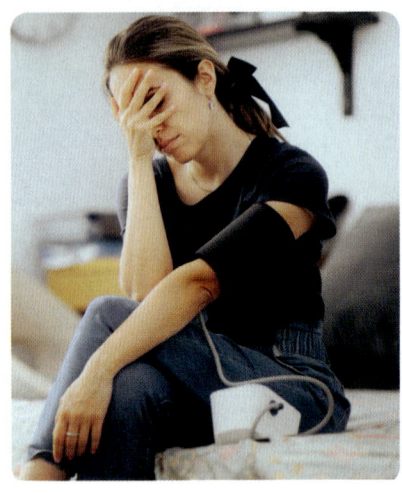

"YOU HAVE THE POWER TO BRING YOUR BLOOD PRESSURE DOWN"

GET YOUR BLOOD PRESSURE CHECKED
There are plenty of options for getting an up-to-date blood pressure reading

If you need to get a current blood pressure reading, then luckily this is quick, easy and free. You may have a machine at home – which you can use to keep an eye on your blood pressure and is discussed earlier in this article – but it's advised to get a reading from someone who is trained, to ensure the accuracy of the numbers. You can usually get a blood pressure check at your normal doctor's surgery, by making an appointment with a doctor or nurse, or there may be a self-service machine in the building. Many pharmacies will offer free checks, as will some gyms and health centres. There are pop-up mobile clinics offering blood pressure checks, and some workplaces will also offer checks. In the UK, NHS Health Checks for those aged between 40 and 74 include blood pressure checks. Should you get a high reading in any location other than a doctor's surgery or hospital, you will need to follow this up with your doctor to discuss next steps or take more readings.

UNDERSTANDING YOUR READINGS
How to put your blood pressure numbers into context

When you have your blood pressure taken, whether by a clinical professional or by yourself at home, you will have two readings, which are displayed one above the other. The top number is your systolic reading in 'mmHG' (millimetres of mercury), and the bottom number is your diastolic reading in mmHG. This will usually be recorded as [top number] / [bottom number] mmHG. If you have your blood pressure taken by a professional, they should give you an indication of whether or not your reading is satisfactory while you are there. However, you may want to know more about your reading and how it sits on a spectrum between low and high blood pressure, or you may have taken a reading yourself and need to put it into context.

Using a chart, like the one seen here, you can plot where your blood pressure is currently at. The systolic reading is tracked on the vertical axis; the diastolic reading on the horizontal. By making a mark where your two readings meet on the chart, you can see visually whereabouts your current blood pressure sits in relation to an optimal blood pressure reading.

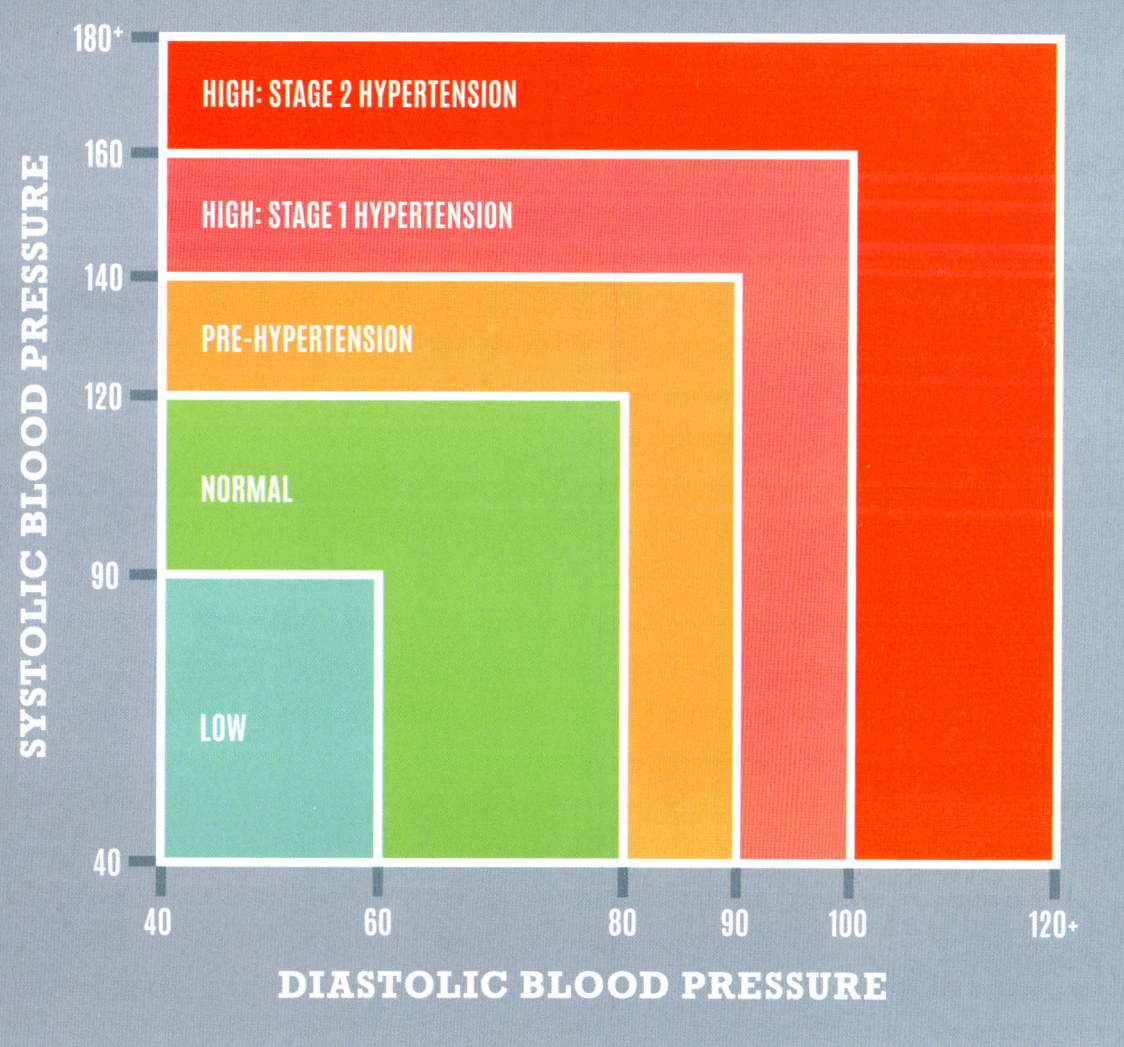

Blood pressure chart

UNDERSTANDING HYPERTENSION

MYTHBUSTING HYPERTENSION

We address the most common misconceptions around high blood pressure

MYTH: HIGH BLOOD PRESSURE ONLY HAPPENS TO OLDER PEOPLE

FACT: You can have high blood pressure at any age, although it is more common in older people due to the natural stiffening of arteries with age. But this can lead to a false sense of security among younger adults who may not consider getting their blood pressure checked regularly. In England, around 7% of men and 4% of women aged 16 to 24 have hypertension[1] and this rises with age, so while it's not really common, it is still a possibility. This is especially true among those with risk factors such as a poor diet high in salt, or excess weight. It's also more likely to be undiagnosed in younger adults.

MYTH: HYPERTENSION IS MORE COMMON IN MEN

FACT: Both men and women are at risk of developing hypertension, though there are some differences between the sexes and the various risk factors. For adults under 50, men are more likely to have high blood pressure than women, which may be linked to a higher prevalence of activities like alcohol or tobacco use. Women are more at risk after menopause, during pregnancy and after taking oral contraceptives. However, there are other risk factors that play a larger role in whether someone develops hypertension.

MYTH: YOU'D KNOW IF YOU HAD HIGH BLOOD PRESSURE

FACT: Quite often, a person can have high blood pressure without any symptoms at all, especially in the early stages. This is why there are so many people who are undiagnosed and why it can lead to serious complications when it's not caught early enough. The only way to know for sure that you have high blood pressure is to have it checked regularly. There are some symptoms that may be noticed in someone with very high blood pressure (which we'll cover later on), but there are rarely noticeable changes in most otherwise healthy people.

MYTH: HIGH BLOOD PRESSURE IS INEVITABLE IF IT RUNS IN THE FAMILY

FACT: Although genetics do play a role in the risk of developing hypertension, it definitely isn't inevitable. It may mean that you could be more prone to developing high blood pressure, but if you adhere to a healthy lifestyle and treatment plan where relevant, you can reverse already existing high blood pressure or prevent it from developing in the first place. This means following a healthy diet, doing regular exercise and getting enough sleep. If you do have a family history of hypertension, then it is even more important to ensure that you have your blood pressure checked regularly.

MYTH: THERE'S NOTHING I CAN DO ABOUT HIGH BLOOD PRESSURE

FACT: It's reassuring to know that you do have quite a lot of control over your high blood pressure. If it's in the early stages, lifestyle intervention can have a huge impact. Quitting smoking, drinking less alcohol and changing your diet can very rapidly start to improve your blood pressure. If you have more severe hypertension, medication can get it under control, while you work on lifestyle changes alongside this to maximise the benefits. It's not a death sentence and you can make a big difference to improving the situation.

[1] ons.gov.uk

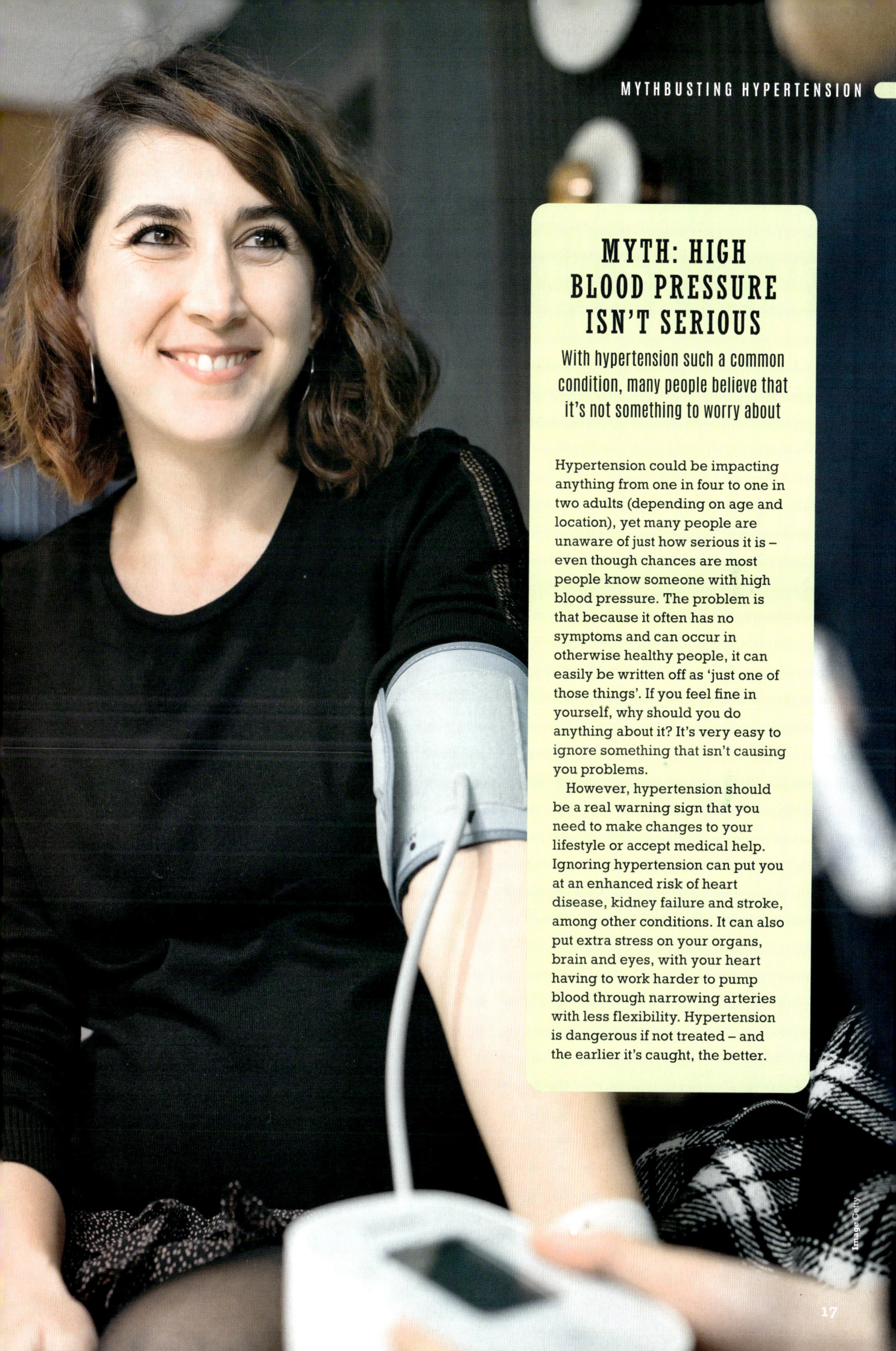

MYTHBUSTING HYPERTENSION

MYTH: HIGH BLOOD PRESSURE ISN'T SERIOUS

With hypertension such a common condition, many people believe that it's not something to worry about

Hypertension could be impacting anything from one in four to one in two adults (depending on age and location), yet many people are unaware of just how serious it is – even though chances are most people know someone with high blood pressure. The problem is that because it often has no symptoms and can occur in otherwise healthy people, it can easily be written off as 'just one of those things'. If you feel fine in yourself, why should you do anything about it? It's very easy to ignore something that isn't causing you problems.

However, hypertension should be a real warning sign that you need to make changes to your lifestyle or accept medical help. Ignoring hypertension can put you at an enhanced risk of heart disease, kidney failure and stroke, among other conditions. It can also put extra stress on your organs, brain and eyes, with your heart having to work harder to pump blood through narrowing arteries with less flexibility. Hypertension is dangerous if not treated – and the earlier it's caught, the better.

UNDERSTANDING HYPERTENSION

WHAT ABOUT CHOLESTEROL?

High cholesterol is linked to high blood pressure, so it's worth knowing your numbers

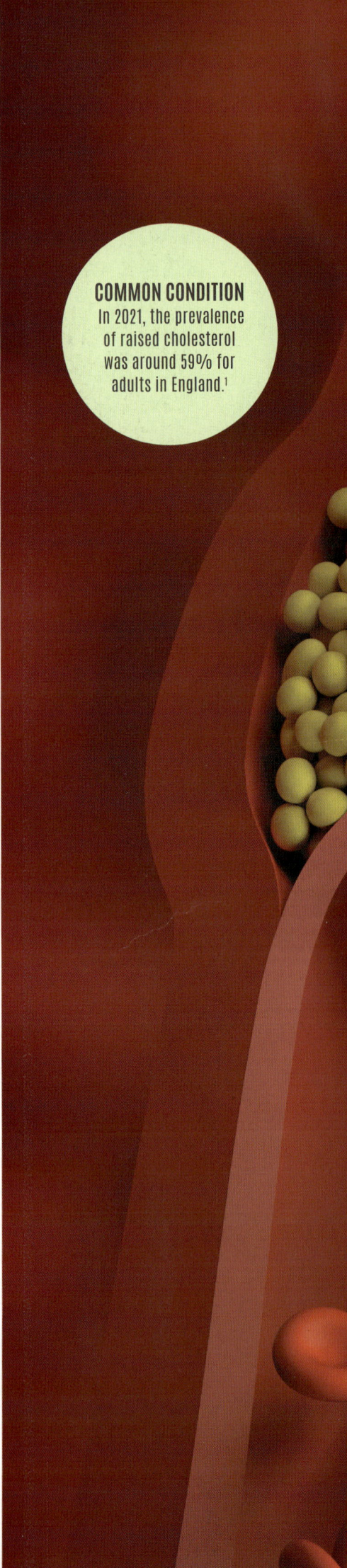

COMMON CONDITION
In 2021, the prevalence of raised cholesterol was around 59% for adults in England.[1]

When you go for a blood pressure reading, you may also be offered a cholesterol check. This is because high cholesterol can block your blood vessels, which can increase your blood pressure. The risk factors are quite similar to hypertension, and the treatment options, such as lifestyle changes, can help reduce both your cholesterol and your blood pressure. Therefore, it's useful to know more about cholesterol and how it's measured.

Cholesterol is a normal part of a healthy body, essential for cell function. It's produced in the liver, but can also be consumed in certain foods. It's a fatty substance that combines with proteins and is transported around your body to your tissues and organs. When cholesterol combines with protein in this way it creates lipoproteins, which come in two main types. The first is non-high-density lipoprotein (non-HDL), and when there is too much of this, it can lead to a build up in your blood vessels, causing them to narrow, which can then increase your blood pressure and your risk of heart attack, heart disease and stroke. And then there is high-density lipoprotein (HDL), which is something that works in a more positive way. It carries non-HDL type cholesterol back to your liver where it can be broken down and removed, rather than letting it build up in your blood. For simplicity, non-HDL is often called the 'bad' cholesterol and HDL is the 'good' cholesterol.

Like high blood pressure, you may not have any symptoms of high cholesterol and the only way to find out is by having a test. This involves taking a small blood sample or finger-prick blood sample. It's a quick process, and you usually get the results straight away if you're having a finger-prick test. The results will show

"ANYONE OF ANY AGE CAN BE DIAGNOSED"

your levels of HDL, non-HDL, and total cholesterol. Ideally you will see a low level of non-HDL and a higher level of HDL. You may also get a reading for triglycerides (see the box on the next page). The person taking your readings should explain if they are in the normal range or not.

Anyone of any age can be diagnosed with high cholesterol, but as with high blood pressure, there are risk factors. In particular, diet can play a big part, especially if you eat a lot of saturated fat. A poor diet can

[1] Health Survey for England 2021, NHS

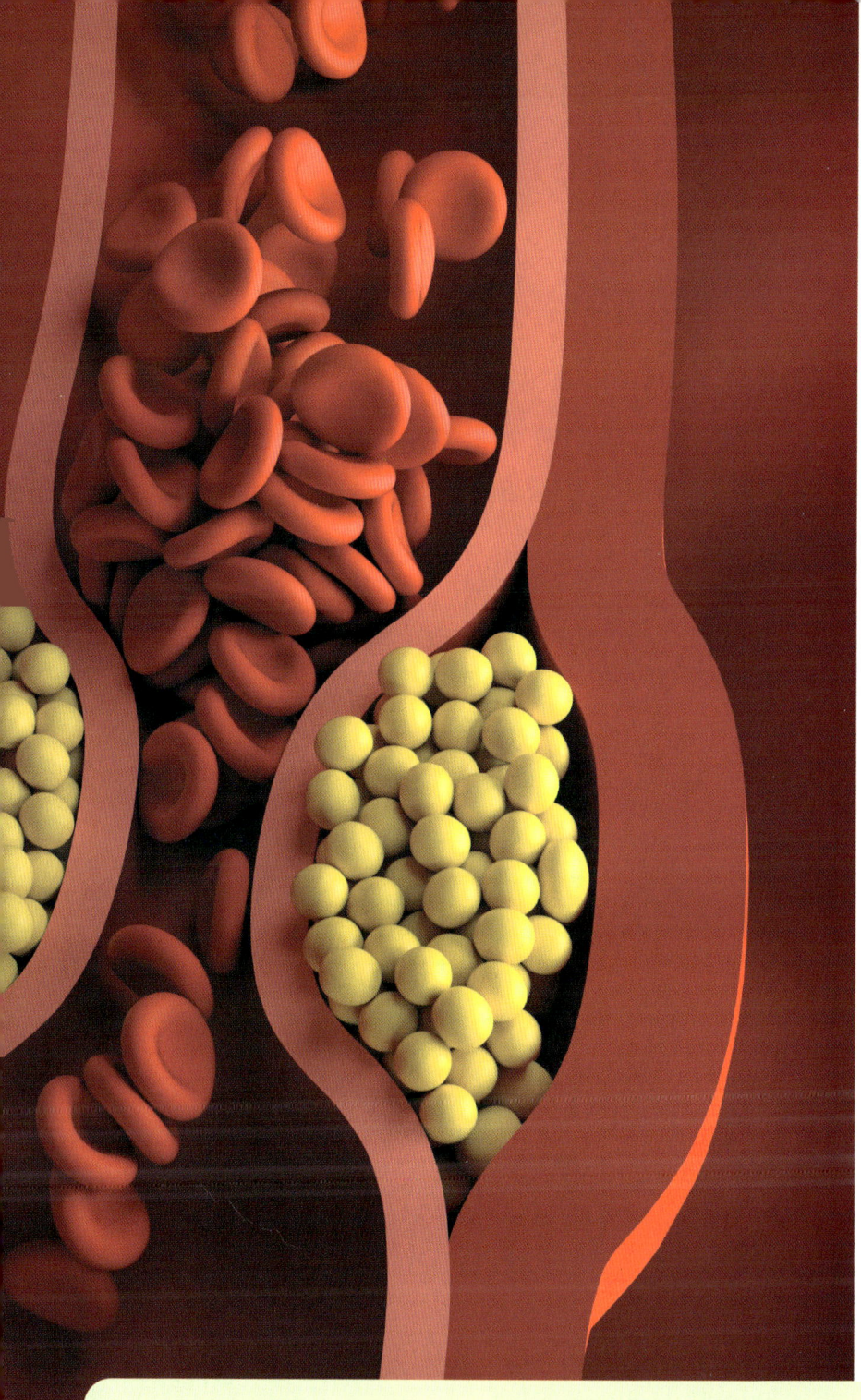

WHAT ABOUT CHOLESTEROL?

make it harder for your liver to remove cholesterol as it should, meaning it builds up in the blood. It's also known that being inactive can impact on cholesterol levels, as can smoking. Other risk factors include being overweight, having type 2 diabetes, having an underactive thyroid or having kidney or liver disease. There are some other risk factors that you can't control, such as age (high cholesterol is more common as you get older), your sex (men are more at risk), and your ethnic background (those from South Asian backgrounds are more at risk). Treatment includes being more physically active, cutting down on alcohol, stopping smoking and eating a healthy balanced diet. There are also medications available for more severe cases.

You can have high cholesterol and low blood pressure, and you can have hypertension with normal levels of cholesterol. However, high cholesterol can contribute to high blood pressure as it narrows the arteries, and high blood pressure can damage the arteries, giving space for cholesterol deposits to build up, so the two are linked. Following the advice for hypertension in this book will also help manage your cholesterol levels.

TRIGLYCERIDES

You may see a reading for this on your cholesterol test, but what is it?

Triglycerides are a type of fat that can be found in your blood, and we need them for energy and healthy cell function. It's the most common type of fat in the body. However, if they build up in the blood, they can cause the arteries to narrow, which can impact on your risk of heart problems. Triglycerides are found in foods like oils, butter and other fatty foods, therefore eating a lot of fatty and sugary foods can lead to excess triglycerides in the blood. Drinking alcohol and being overweight can also cause this type of fat to build up.

If your triglyceride level is found to be high, you will be advised to follow a healthy diet and be physically active to help bring these levels down. You can have high triglycerides but normal cholesterol levels, which is why a full profile from your blood is useful, and there is some research that suggests a link between high triglycerides and hypertension.

UNDERSTANDING
HYPERTENSION

CAUSES AND RISK FACTORS

Hypertension is caused by many different things, and some of us are more at risk than others

Finding out you have hypertension can be worrying, especially knowing it can be a major risk factor for serious conditions and complications. Upon diagnosis, people often want to know what has caused it so they can take steps to resolve the problem, but in most cases, there isn't a single or specific reason why you have high blood pressure. It is often a combination of factors, some that are controllable and others that aren't. However, knowing the possible causes and risk factors of hypertension can help you identify the key areas you might need to target when it comes to making lifestyle changes, for example.

In some cases of hypertension there is a cause, where high blood pressure has been influenced by another health condition or by medications. In these cases, it is called 'secondary hypertension', and we'll cover this in its own feature. Here we'll look at why hypertension can occur without a specific underlying reason.

LIFESTYLE RISK FACTORS

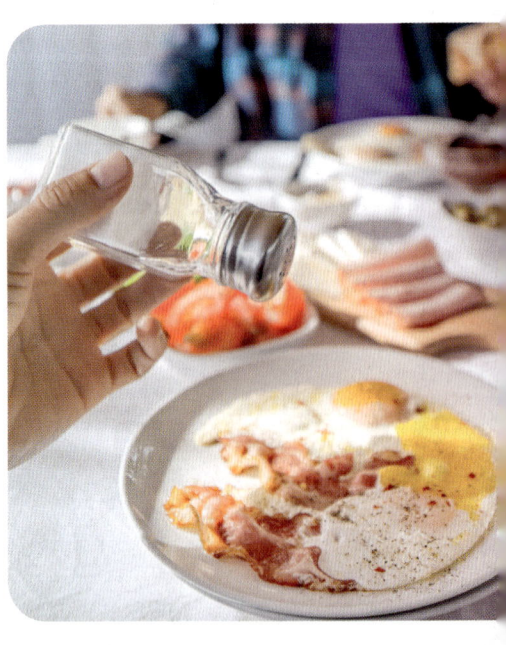

The way you live your life can have a big impact on your risk of developing hypertension. In particular, what you eat can directly affect your blood pressure. If your diet is high in salt, this can contribute to hypertension; adults should have no more than six grams of salt a day, which is about a teaspoon. The problem is that salt is hidden in lots of everyday foods, so it's easy to eat too much of it without realising. Salt causes the body to retain more fluid, and this extra fluid can lead to more water passing through the blood vessels, putting pressure on them and therefore increasing your blood pressure. In fact, according to bloodpressureuk.org, eating too much salt is the single biggest cause of high blood pressure, and addressing this can have a fast impact on your readings.

As well as salt, other aspects of your diet can contribute to high blood pressure. If you eat a lot of ultra-processed foods high in sugar and fat, you may find it harder to maintain a healthy weight – a key lifestyle risk factor.

Carrying excess weight can also be a significant contributing factor towards hypertension. When you have a higher body weight, your heart has to work harder to pump blood around the body, raising

CAUSES AND RISK FACTORS

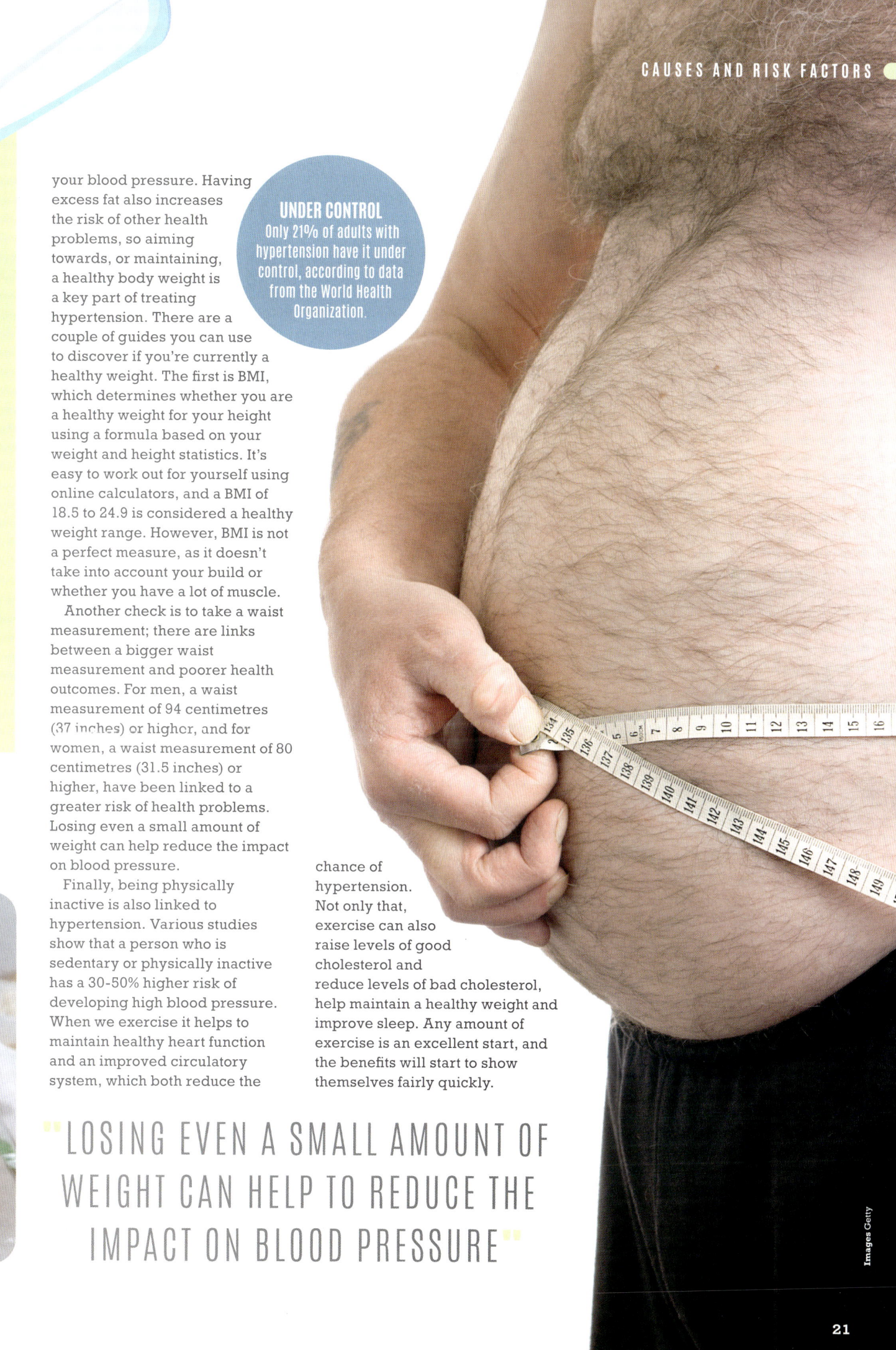

your blood pressure. Having excess fat also increases the risk of other health problems, so aiming towards, or maintaining, a healthy body weight is a key part of treating hypertension. There are a couple of guides you can use to discover if you're currently a healthy weight. The first is BMI, which determines whether you are a healthy weight for your height using a formula based on your weight and height statistics. It's easy to work out for yourself using online calculators, and a BMI of 18.5 to 24.9 is considered a healthy weight range. However, BMI is not a perfect measure, as it doesn't take into account your build or whether you have a lot of muscle.

Another check is to take a waist measurement; there are links between a bigger waist measurement and poorer health outcomes. For men, a waist measurement of 94 centimetres (37 inches) or higher, and for women, a waist measurement of 80 centimetres (31.5 inches) or higher, have been linked to a greater risk of health problems. Losing even a small amount of weight can help reduce the impact on blood pressure.

Finally, being physically inactive is also linked to hypertension. Various studies show that a person who is sedentary or physically inactive has a 30-50% higher risk of developing high blood pressure. When we exercise it helps to maintain healthy heart function and an improved circulatory system, which both reduce the chance of hypertension. Not only that, exercise can also raise levels of good cholesterol and reduce levels of bad cholesterol, help maintain a healthy weight and improve sleep. Any amount of exercise is an excellent start, and the benefits will start to show themselves fairly quickly.

> **UNDER CONTROL**
> Only 21% of adults with hypertension have it under control, according to data from the World Health Organization.

"LOSING EVEN A SMALL AMOUNT OF WEIGHT CAN HELP TO REDUCE THE IMPACT ON BLOOD PRESSURE"

UNDERSTANDING HYPERTENSION

SUBSTANCE USE

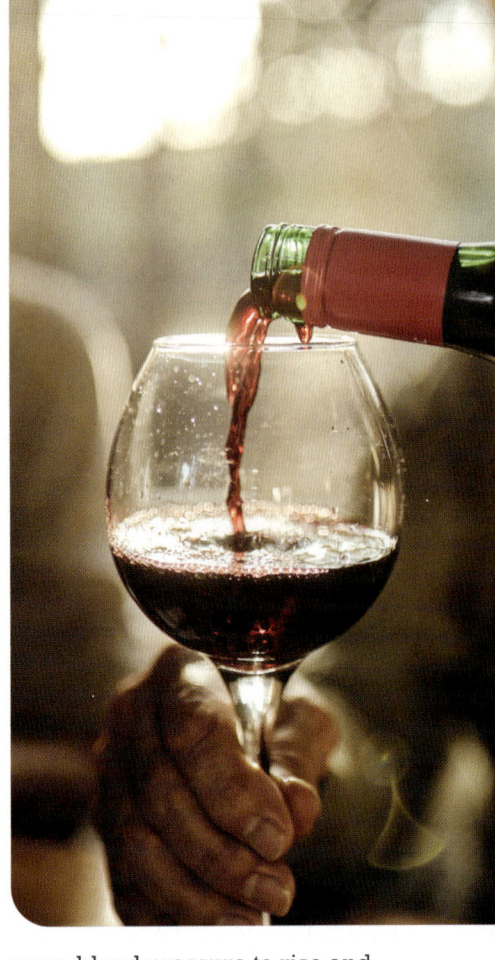

Certain substances can directly impact your risk of developing hypertension. One of the biggest factors is whether you smoke or not. Smoking just one cigarette causes a short-term rise in blood pressure, so if you're having numerous cigarettes per day, you are likely to have consistently high blood pressure. Plus, the toxins in a cigarette directly damage the walls of blood vessels and cause fatty buildups that narrow the blood vessels, and they can also make your blood more likely to clot. All of this forces your heart to work harder to pump blood around the body, increasing the risk of heart attack and stroke. Smoking also causes a huge number of other health problems, so giving up smoking can have significant benefits to your overall health.

Alcohol is another contributing factor when it comes to hypertension. If you drink more than the recommended amount on a regular basis, you may develop high blood pressure. Like cigarettes, even a single drink raises blood pressure in the short term, so if you don't give your body a break between drinks or drinking sessions, it can lead to sustained high blood pressure. Drinking excessive amounts of alcohol also leads to other health complications and conditions, so it's advised to cut down or stop drinking to help treat high blood pressure. The current guidelines in the UK are to drink no more than 14 units a week, spread out over the week, and with alcohol-free days in between. However, if you already have hypertension, you may be advised to keep to a much lower amount.

Recreational illegal drugs are a known contributor to hypertension as well. Most common drugs will cause blood pressure to rise and the heart to pump faster, which over time can lead to serious problems. Some substances, like cocaine, will directly narrow the blood vessels, increasing their pressure, as well as causing damage to cardiac tissue.

It's often been thought that caffeine has a big impact on blood pressure, but most research shows that a moderate amount of tea or coffee each day is fine for most people and shouldn't directly affect your blood pressure, heart function or cholesterol. While drinking caffeine can cause a temporary increase in blood pressure, this should pass, especially if you drink caffeine

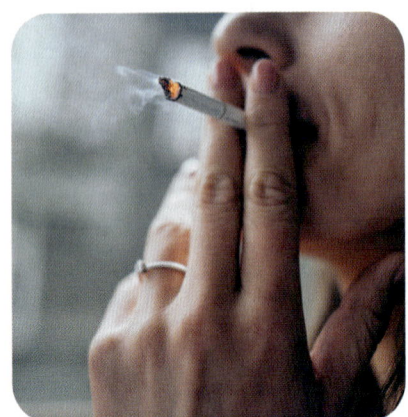

WHAT ABOUT STRESS?
Many of us think of stress and blood pressure as being linked, but are they?

We often think of stress as being a reason why we might have high blood pressure. A short-term rise in blood pressure in response to stress is a normal reaction. It's part of our fight-or-flight response to a perceived threat, with the body releasing more adrenaline and raising the heart rate to help us manage what we're dealing with. Once the stress has passed, blood pressure should return to normal. Stress alone isn't a cause for hypertension.

However, sustained levels of stress over the long term can lead to us indulging in unhealthy habits that can increase the risk for high blood pressure. This includes things like eating too much unhealthy food, smoking, drinking more than usual or not finding time for regular exercise. This is why it's beneficial to learn to manage stress and to make lifestyle changes that help to keep stress under control for overall health and wellbeing.

CAUSES AND RISK FACTORS

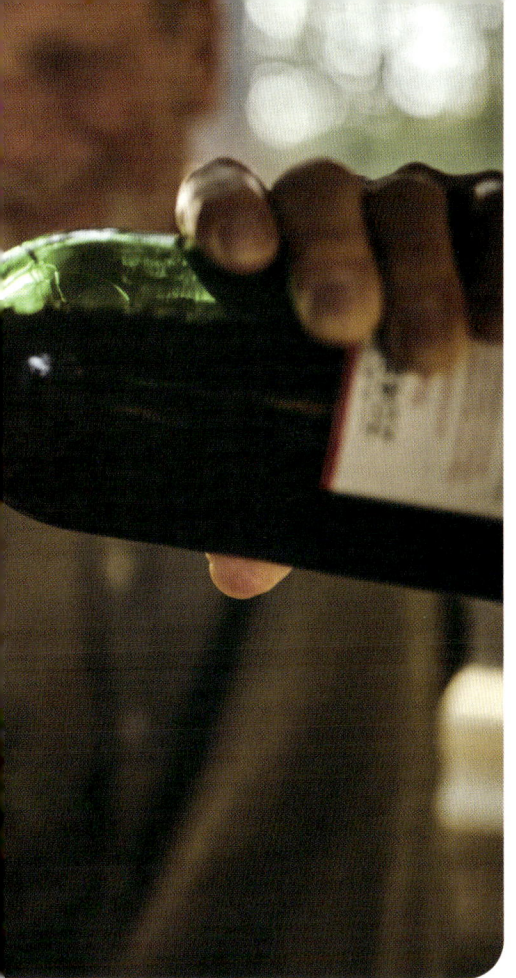

> "MOST COMMON DRUGS WILL CAUSE BLOOD PRESSURE TO RISE"

UNDIAGNOSED HYPERTENSION RISK

If you don't know you have high blood pressure, this puts you at more risk of complications

Once you have been diagnosed with hypertension, you can start to do something about it. The problem is that many people don't know about it, which means there is the risk that it can get worse; by the time a person is diagnosed, it's already at a more severe stage. Catching hypertension as early as possible means that it can be monitored and treated to prevent it from getting any worse. There are lots of research studies that have tried to put a figure on the number of undiagnosed adults, however these are estimates as there are some countries and demographics where there are gaps in prevention, monitoring and treatment. The World Health Organization estimates around 580 million people with hypertension are unaware of their condition, despite the fact that it's easy to diagnose and the treatments available are low in cost and accessible. This is why many countries have introduced age-related check-ups in order to catch hypertension as early as possible.

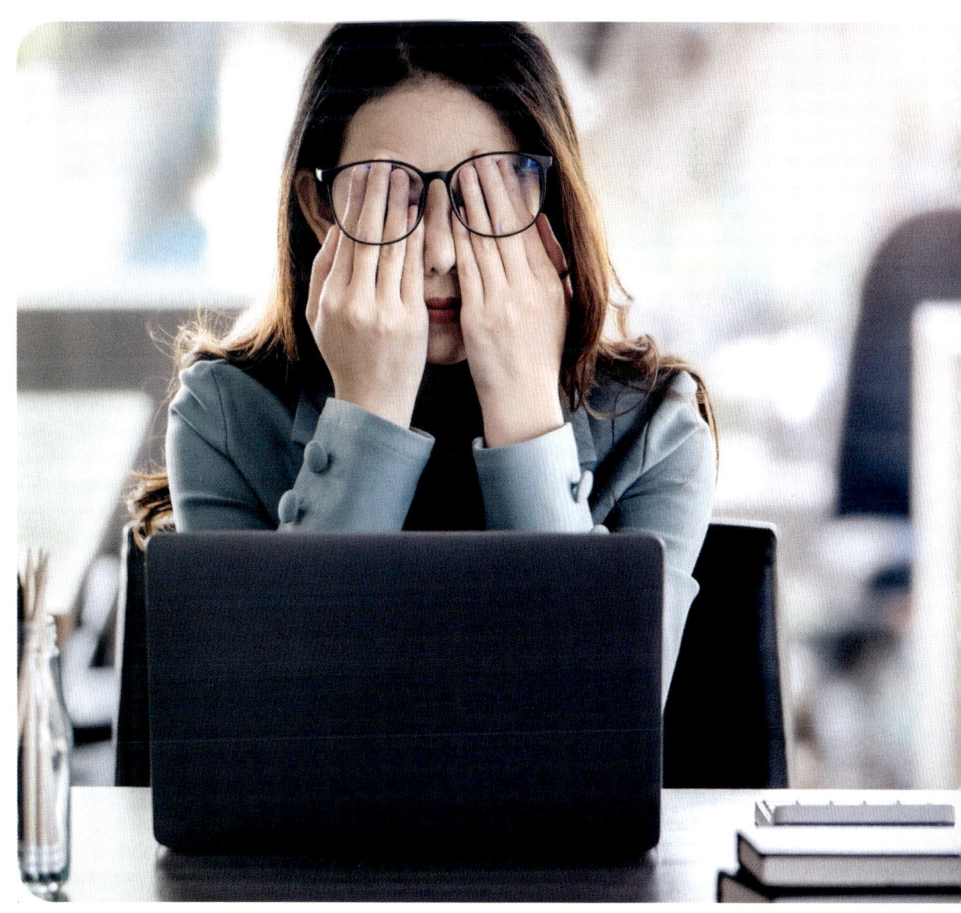

regularly and you're not overly sensitive to it. A moderate amount of caffeine is usually considered to be between four and five cups per day. What can be more significant, however, is how you take your tea or coffee. If you're adding sugar, cream, a lot of milk or syrups, for example, then this can contribute to weight gain or higher cholesterol levels, which can then have a knock-on effect on your blood pressure. Also, don't forget that caffeine can be found in other foods and drinks, such as soft drinks, energy drinks and chocolate, and these should all be considered when monitoring your daily caffeine intake.

UNDERSTANDING
HYPERTENSION

UNMODIFIABLE CAUSES

There are some causes and risk factors of hypertension that you can't do anything about. First, your risk of hypertension increases with age. About 5% of people aged 16 to 24 years (in England, but the figure is similar worldwide) have high blood pressure, but this rises to over half (58%) at 65 to 75. This is partly due to the natural process of arteries narrowing and getting stiffer over time, but it could also be a culminative effect of unhealthy lifestyle choices or increasing weight as we age. We may also be more likely to have other health conditions with age that can be linked to high blood pressure, or be taking medications that contribute to hypertension. However, even in the older age categories, making lifestyle changes can reduce blood pressure.

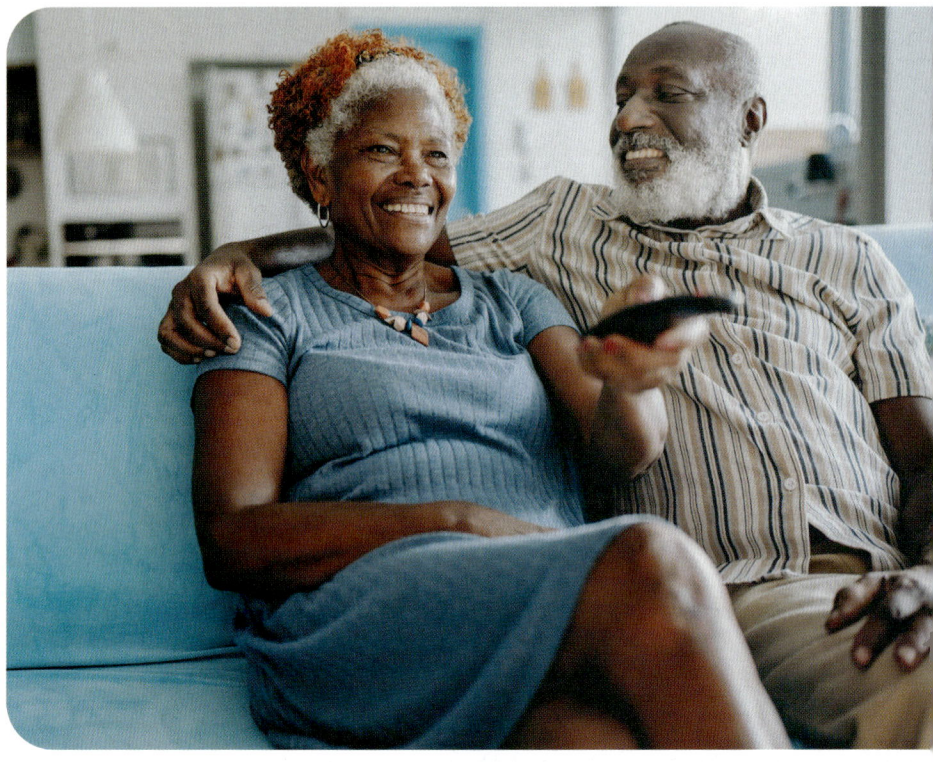

We're also learning more about the role genetics play in the development of hypertension. If someone in your family has had high blood pressure, you're at an increased risk of developing it yourself. There's nothing you can do about your genetics, but if you know your family is prone to high blood pressure, you can make lifestyle changes to reduce your risk. A 2021 study from the University of Manchester, supported by the British Heart Foundation and Kidney Research UK, discovered 179 kidney genes responsible for high blood pressure, of which around 80% had never been associated with blood pressure before. This sort of research may lead to new treatments being used to help lower and control hypertension.

Sex and gender are also risk factors for blood pressure, however both sexes are at higher risk at different points in their lives. A low-risk man is more likely to develop hypertension than a low-risk woman over a lifetime, and men have a higher prevalence of hypertension as younger adults. However, there are risk factors that only impact women, such as pregnancy, going through or having gone through menopause, and using hormonal contraceptives. The risk of high blood pressure in women rises rapidly with age to the point at

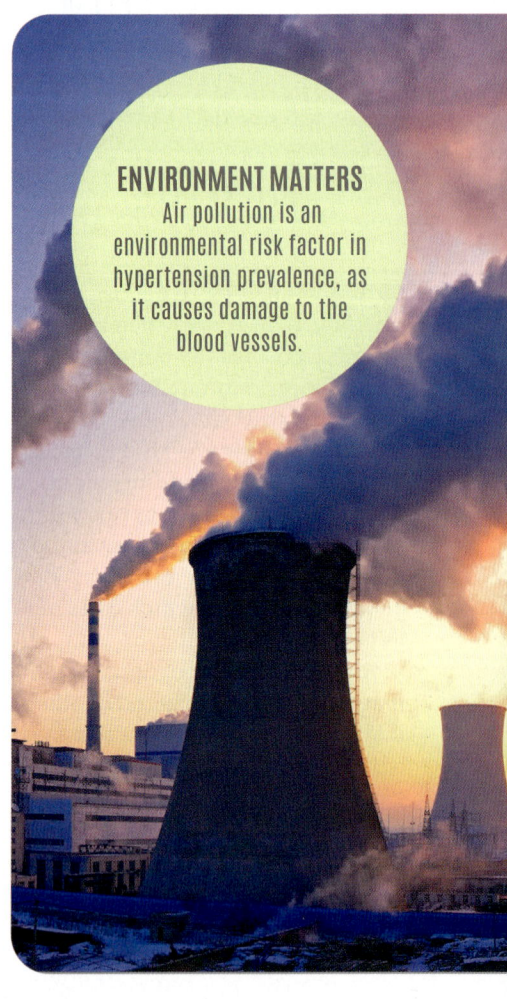

ENVIRONMENT MATTERS
Air pollution is an environmental risk factor in hypertension prevalence, as it causes damage to the blood vessels.

> "THERE'S NOTHING YOU CAN DO ABOUT YOUR GENETICS"

CAUSES AND RISK FACTORS

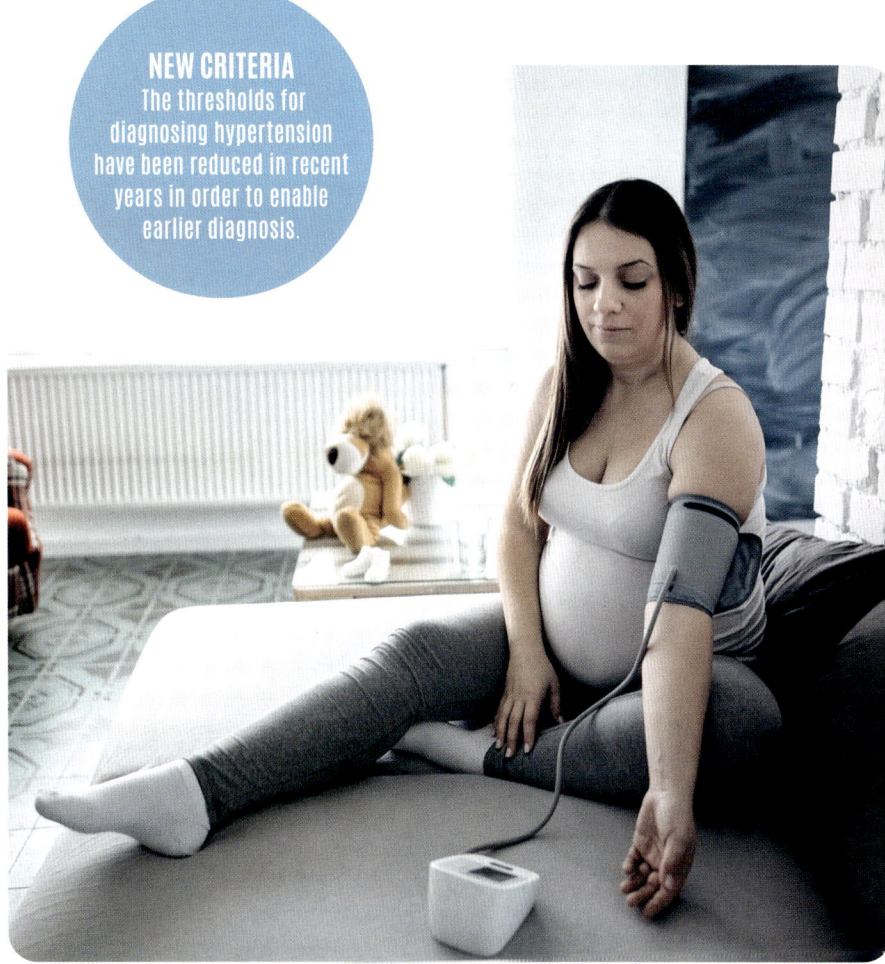

NEW CRITERIA
The thresholds for diagnosing hypertension have been reduced in recent years in order to enable earlier diagnosis.

which the risk becomes greater than men.

Race and ethnicity also impact the risk of high blood pressure. A health survey from 2022 (NHS England) found a marked variance in hypertension among different ethnic groups, even when standardised for age. Those of Black Caribbean, Black African or Pakistani heritage had the highest prevalence of hypertension, and it may develop at a younger age.

There are also socioeconomic risk factors. Those on a lower income are shown to be more likely to develop hypertension, as are those who left education at an earlier stage. Environmental risk factors based on location, as well as occupational factors can also contribute to increased risk.

As you can see, there are many factors that contribute to whether a person develops hypertension or not. It can therefore be more proactive to focus on treatment and prevention, rather than cause.

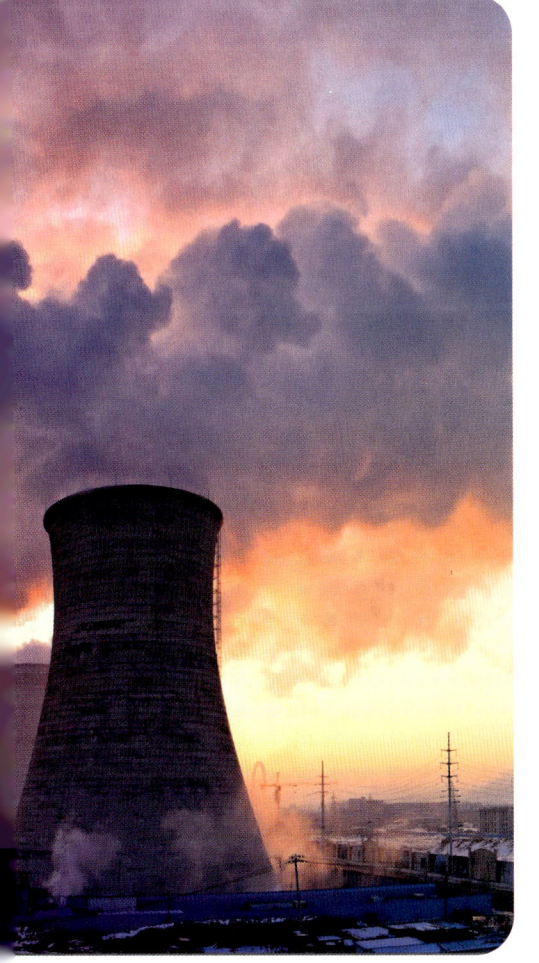

HYPERTENSION IN PREGNANCY
Women can be more at risk of high blood pressure when pregnant

Women who are pregnant will have their blood pressure checked more regularly, one of the reasons being because having hypertension can sometimes be more serious in pregnancy. If a problem is found, how it's dealt with will depend on whether it's mild, moderate or severe, and whether it's newly developed in pregnancy or something that was diagnosed previously.

Those who have a history of high blood pressure will usually be referred to a specialist during the pregnancy. Some medicines that are normally used to treat hypertension are not suitable for use in pregnancy due to the fact that they can reduce blood flow to the placenta. In these circumstances, lifestyle changes can help, including staying active and eating a healthy, balanced diet. Some women may develop pre-eclampsia, which is a problem with the placenta that can cause blood pressure to rise, and is more common in those who have had high blood pressure before becoming pregnant. This is a serious condition if left untreated, so it's important to have all the checks that are offered.

UNDERSTANDING HYPERTENSION

SECONDARY HYPERTENSION

We explore other health conditions or causes that can lead to elevated blood pressure

GET ADVICE
If you're concerned about secondary hypertension, speak to your care team about what you can do to get it under control.

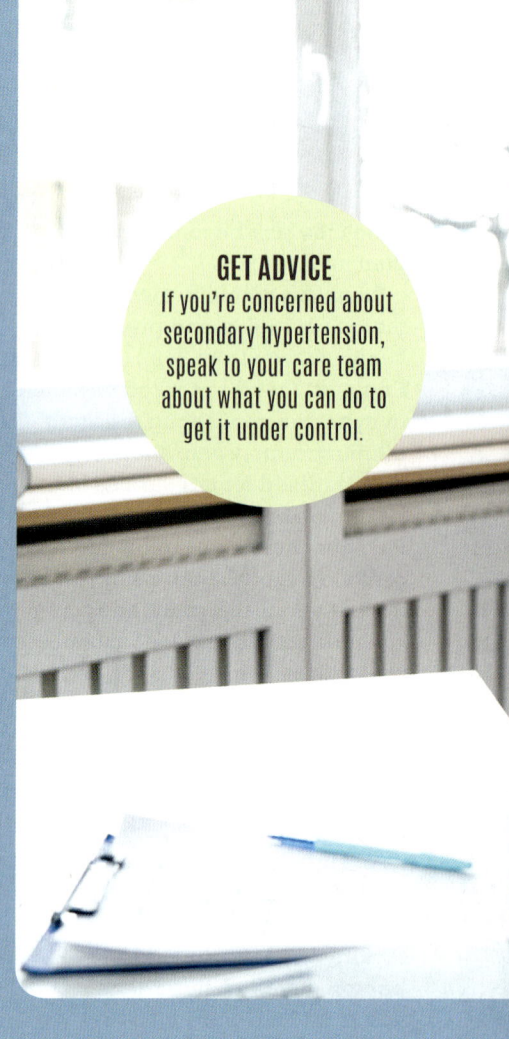

For most people, there is no single cause for hypertension; rather a combination of lifestyle, genetic and environmental factors. However, in some cases, hypertension is caused by another health condition or by certain medications. This is called secondary hypertension. It's not a common condition, impacting around 5% of all people diagnosed with hypertension.

As it's a secondary diagnosis, it can be found in younger people as well as older people; in fact, one figure[1] suggests that in young adults under 40, the prevalence of secondary hypertension is about 30% (remember that those in this age range are at a lower risk of primary hypertension). Secondary hypertension might be indicated in circumstances where a person is diagnosed at a younger age, has no excess weight or has no family history, or where blood pressure doesn't respond to the usual high blood pressure medication. All of these can be signs that there is an underlying reason for the hypertension. The most common factors that can cause secondary hypertension are kidney conditions or endocrine system conditions, however there are other conditions, such as diabetes, that are sometimes linked with (although not direct causes of) high blood pressure.

In these pages we will look at some of the common conditions linked with hypertension, however there are many more and this is something that will be shared with you if you are diagnosed with a health condition that impacts blood pressure.

Kidney disease

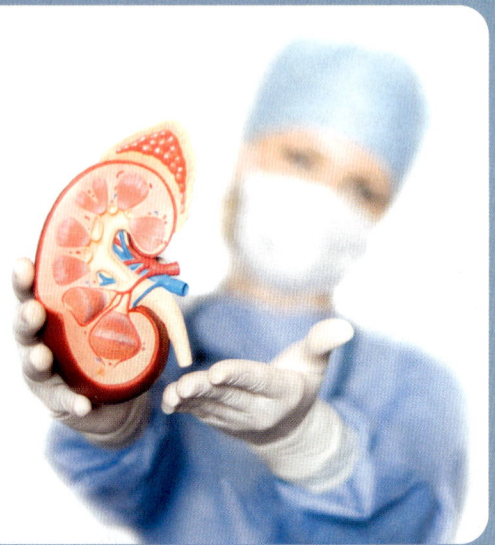

Chronic kidney disease (CKD) is a long-term condition that is more common in older adults over 65, though it can affect people of all ages. It's also more common in people who are Black or of South Asian origin. CKD can be both a direct cause of hypertension or a consequence of it. The early stages of CKD have few, if any, symptoms, so it often doesn't get picked up until a much later stage. It tends to only be caught earlier if a blood or urine test is performed for another reason. It can get worse over time, though many people can control it with medicine, lifestyle changes and regular check-ups.

Healthy kidneys play a key role when it comes to regulating blood pressure. This means that if someone's kidneys are damaged, it can have a knock-on effect on elevating blood pressure. As hypertension can cause more damage to the kidneys, it's easy to get stuck in a cycle of one impacting the other. Sometimes it can be difficult to tell if primary hypertension has caused the kidney disease, or if the kidney disease has led to secondary hypertension. Therefore, it's really important

SECONDARY HYPERTENSION

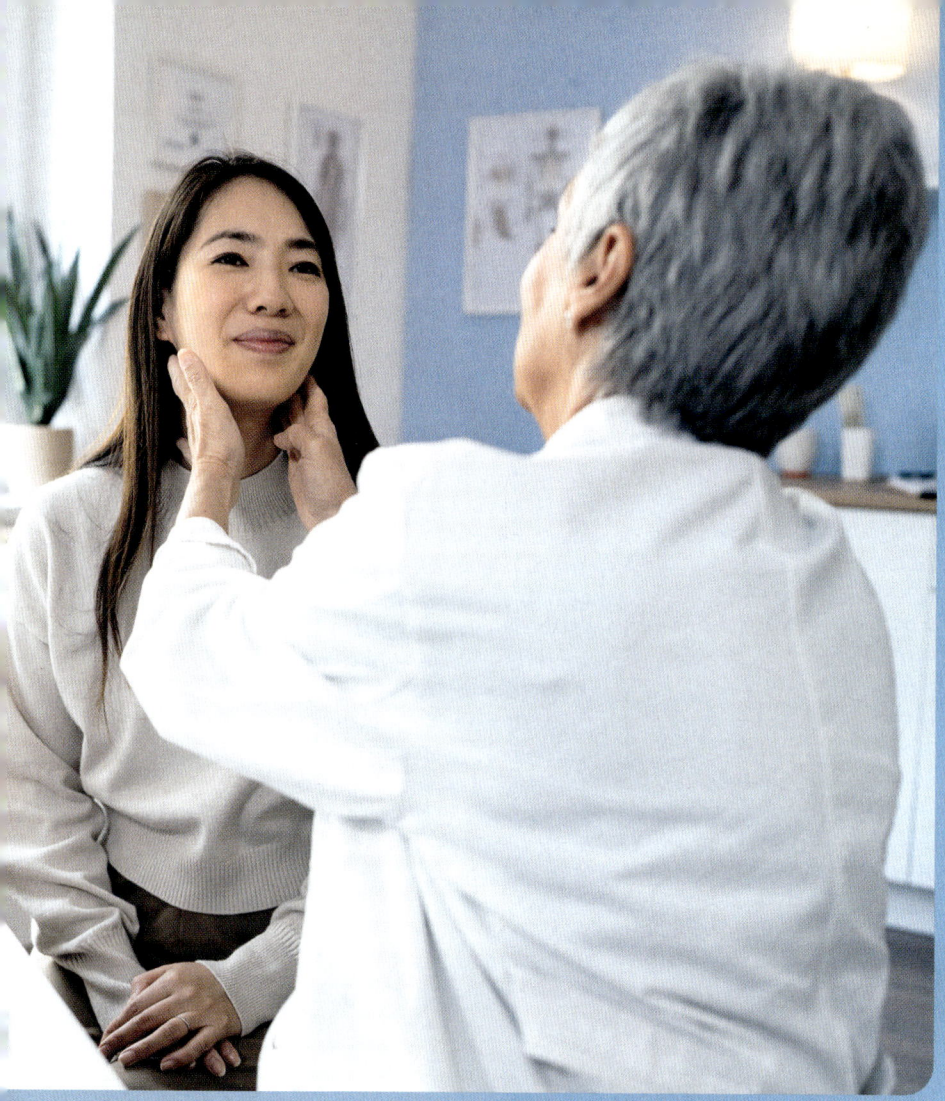

> "AN UNDERACTIVE THYROID CAN ALSO SLOW DOWN THE HEART"

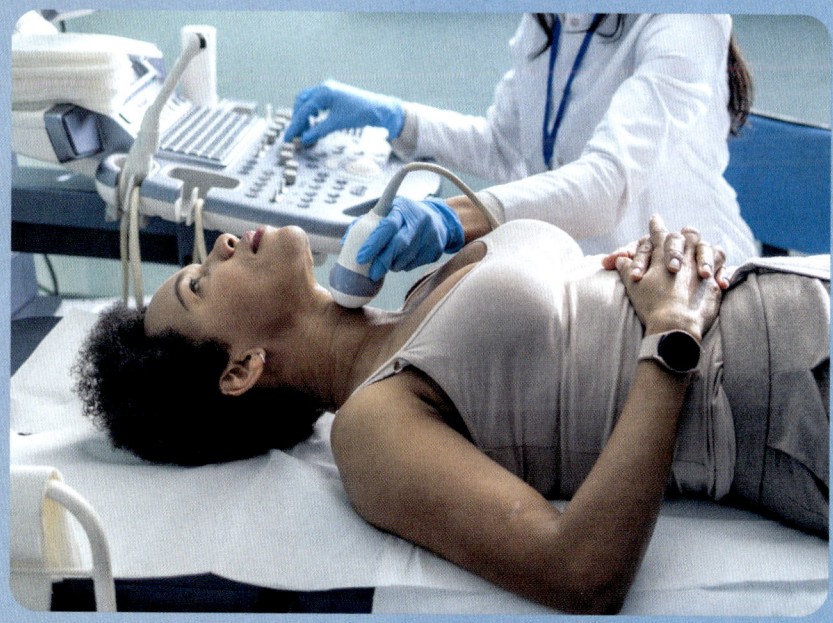

to treat both CKD and the resulting hypertension to prevent further health complications. Luckily, the main lifestyle interventions for hypertension can also help with the kidney disease, including following a healthy low-salt diet, exercising regularly, not smoking and limiting alcohol.

There is also autosomal dominant polycystic kidney disease (ADPKD), which is an inherited condition causing cysts to develop in the kidneys. While people are born with the condition, it doesn't usually cause problems until the cysts grow larger, which usually happens after the age of 30. One of the consequences of ADPKD at this more advanced stage is secondary hypertension. It's a relatively uncommon condition with no cure, but it can be managed through a healthy lifestyle and specific treatments to manage the various related problems.

Endocrine disorders

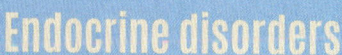

The endocrine system refers to the glands and organs that make hormones, and there are various disorders and conditions that can impact this delicate system. Some of these will have a knock-on effect on blood pressure.

For example, if thyroid function is disrupted, this can lead to secondary hypertension. Hypothyroidism (an underactive thyroid) is when the thyroid gland doesn't produce enough hormones for your body. One of the consequences of an underactive thyroid is that the lack of hormones can change the way the body processes fat, which can increase the cholesterol levels in your blood. This can then cause fatty deposits to build up in your blood, restricting blood flow and increasing blood pressure. An underactive thyroid can also slow down the heart, which means it

UNDERSTANDING HYPERTENSION

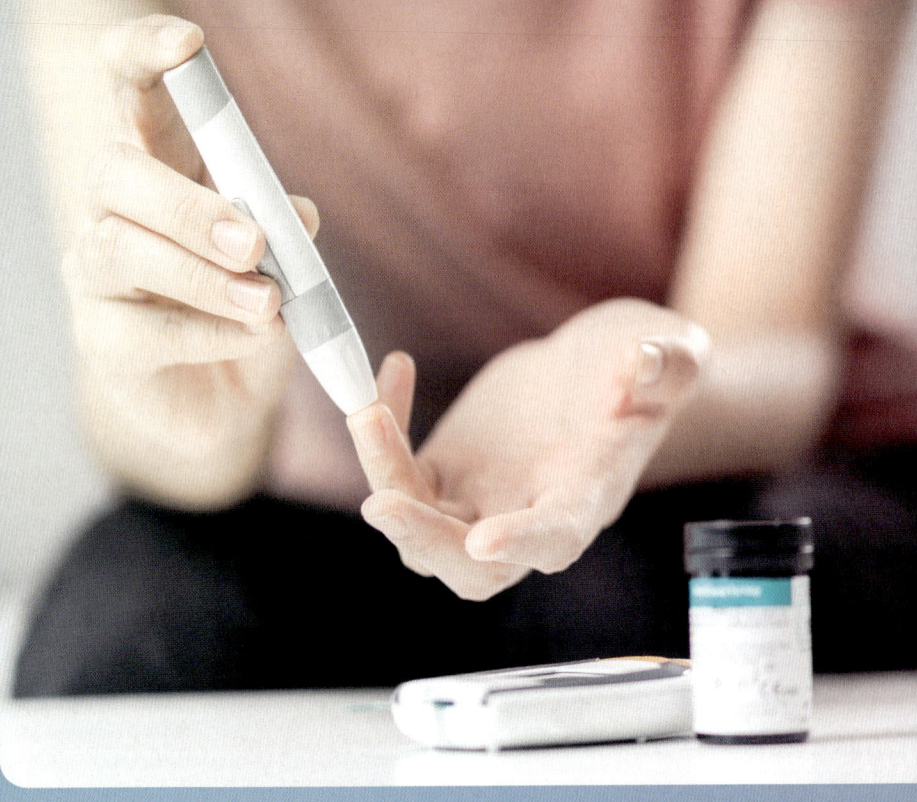

has to work harder to pump blood around the body, also causing a rise in blood pressure.

An overactive thyroid (hyperthyroidism) can also cause secondary hypertension, sometimes making the heart work harder and leading to an increase in systolic pressure. Treatment for hyperthyroidism can sometimes lead to hypothyroidism and the related consequences of that. Undiagnosed or poorly controlled hyperthyroidism can lead to a serious complication called a 'thyroid storm', one of the symptoms of which is – you guessed it – high blood pressure.

Cushing's syndrome is a condition related to unbalanced hormone levels, caused by having too much cortisol in the body. It's not a very common condition, usually experienced in those who have been taking steroid medicine for a long time. On rare occasions, it can be caused by the body producing too much cortisol due to a benign tumour in the pituitary gland in the brain, or the adrenal glands near the kidneys. Cushing's syndrome can cause secondary hypertension.

Diabetes

If someone has diabetes, then it's standard to take a blood pressure reading as part of their normal regular check-ups. Diabetes is when blood sugar levels are too high due to not making enough, or becoming resistant to, insulin. The high levels of blood sugar in uncontrolled diabetes can cause a number of complications, including damage to your blood vessels and problems with your kidneys. Having diabetes increases your risk of heart disease and stroke.

There are two main types of diabetes. Type 1 diabetes usually develops at a young age and can't be prevented; the body doesn't produce insulin and this needs to be managed through insulin injections. Type 2 diabetes is when the body stops making enough insulin or the body becomes resistant to it. This is far more common than type 1 diabetes and is often linked to being overweight, inactive or unhealthy. There are other risk factors for developing diabetes, including ethnicity, age, family history and high blood pressure.

Much like hypertension, diabetes doesn't have many symptoms in the early stages. However, the high blood sugar levels can be causing serious problems without you realising. Your blood vessels can become damaged, leading to fatty deposits

"HAVING MORE THAN ONE CONDITION INCREASES THE RISK OF HEART DISEASE"

building up in your arteries, causing them to narrow. This can lead to elevated blood pressure because the arteries are under more strain. Having diabetes doesn't directly cause hypertension and vice versa, but they share many similarities in terms of risk factors. And having more than one condition at the same time further increases the risk of heart disease and stroke.

For those who already have diabetes, it's important to keep an eye on blood pressure and, where necessary, take medications that will help to lower blood pressure closer to the healthy range. Some medications for high blood pressure might not be suitable for those with diabetes, so it's important to work with a doctor to find the right treatment. Lifestyle interventions are incredibly important, as they help to manage both blood pressure and the diabetes itself.

While this book mainly focuses on primary hypertension, the treatments and interventions are just as relevant for secondary hypertension. However, if you have an underlying condition, any changes should be made in conjunction with your care team. If you have any concerns about underlying conditions or your health, you should always speak to a doctor.

SECONDARY HYPERTENSION

MEDICATIONS

Hypertension can be a side effect of some commonly used medicines

Some medicines can make blood pressure medication less effective, and others can make it harder to lower your blood pressure through lifestyle changes. There are even medications, as well as herbal remedies, that can directly cause your blood pressure to rise – always read the leaflets that come with medicines to be sure.

Ibuprofen, for example, can create a rise in blood pressure as it causes blood vessels to narrow. Those who have high blood pressure that's not under control are usually advised not to take it. This is also true of decongestants, which are designed to help clear a blocked or stuffy nose. The way they work is by reducing inflammation in the nose, but this also causes blood vessels to narrow, which can increase blood pressure. Anyone with high blood pressure should seek advice from a doctor before using a decongestant. You should also be aware of any medications that can't be combined. In this case, taking a decongestant alongside some antidepressants can cause a dangerous rise in blood pressure.

ST JOHN'S WORT
This herbal remedy, used to help with mental health conditions, can react with some blood pressure medications.

Oral contraceptive pills have been known to cause high blood pressure in some people, though this is more likely to happen in people who have other risk factors, such as being overweight, being a smoker, being older or having a family history of hypertension. Certain antidepressants, in particular SNRIs (serotonin and norepinephrine reuptake inhibitors), are not always suitable for people with hypertension that's not currently under control.

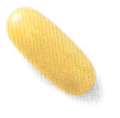
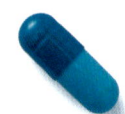

SLEEP APNOEA

Hypertension can be linked to this sleep disorder

Obstructive sleep apnoea (OSA) is a condition where a person's breathing stops and starts when asleep. The affected person may make gasping or choking noises at night, snore loudly, or audibly stop breathing momentarily before starting again. This can lead to waking up a lot at night, feeling very tired, and finding it difficult to focus the next day. Quite often it's someone else who notices that a person has the condition, as obviously most of the symptoms happen when the affected person is asleep.

Sleep apnoea can lead to other complications, one of which is high blood pressure. According to sleepfoundation.org, the prevalence of OSA in the USA is about 4-7% in the general population, but affects 30-40% of people with hypertension; and of those diagnosed with OSA, around half have hypertension. It's thought this link is because disturbed sleep affects normal blood pressure function. For most of us, blood pressure naturally dips at night, but in those with OSA this might not happen. They may also experience a sudden surge in blood pressure in the morning, as well as sustained elevation of blood pressure in the daytime. The body is essentially under stress throughout the night, which can raise the heart rate and blood pressure.

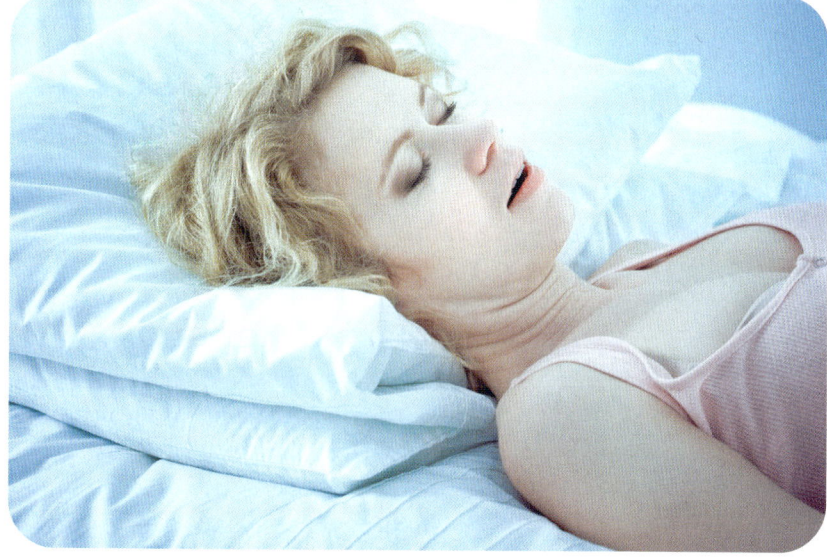

UNDERSTANDING
HYPERTENSION

RISKS AND HEALTH IMPLICATIONS

Having high blood pressure puts you at a bigger risk of health complications. We look at the most serious conditions

High blood pressure can be easy to ignore, especially as it has no noticeable symptoms for most people, particularly in the early stages. However, it is a dangerous thing to leave untreated, as it can progress in severity and possibly lead to some very serious health complications. Therefore, if you're told that you have high blood pressure, no matter what stage it is at, you should start to take measures to help get it under control as soon as you can.

In this feature, we'll talk about the biggest risks of having hypertension. However, don't let it worry you too much, as you can start to make changes as soon as you're diagnosed and begin to lower your risk.

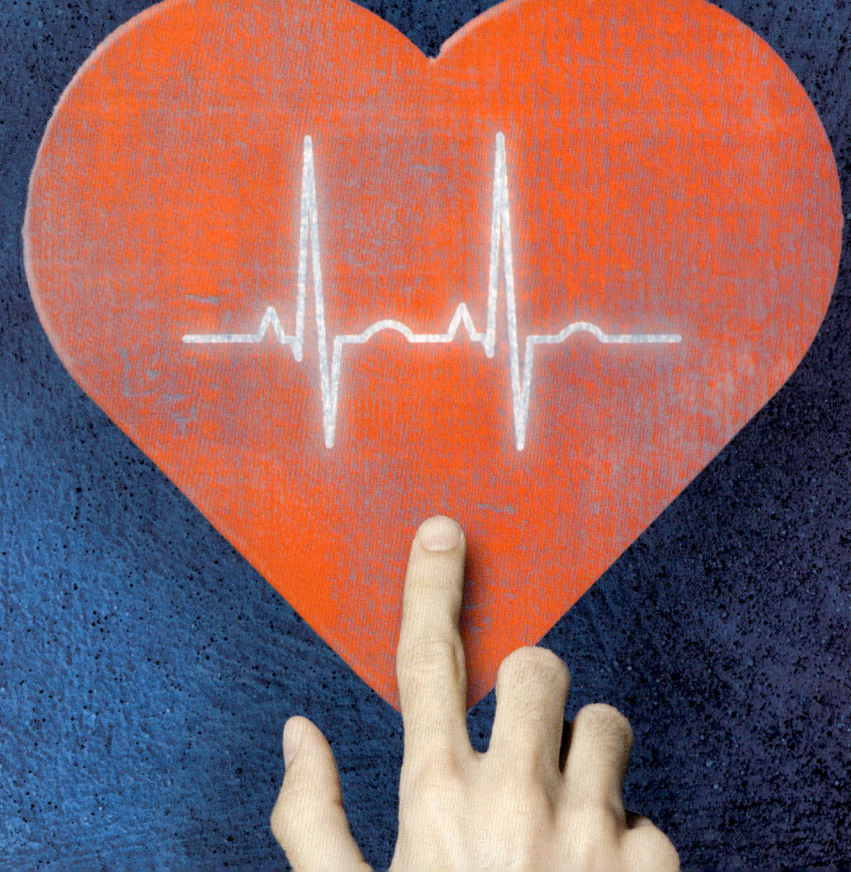

RISKS AND HEALTH IMPLICATIONS

RISK OF HEART CONDITIONS

One of the biggest concerns when it comes to hypertension is that it can contribute to your risk of developing cardiovascular diseases (CVDs). This is a general term referring to several conditions that affect the heart or blood vessels. CVDs are the leading cause of death globally – in 2019, almost 18 million people died from CVDs, which was about a third of all global deaths[1]. While there are many different types of CVD, some of the most serious are heart conditions.

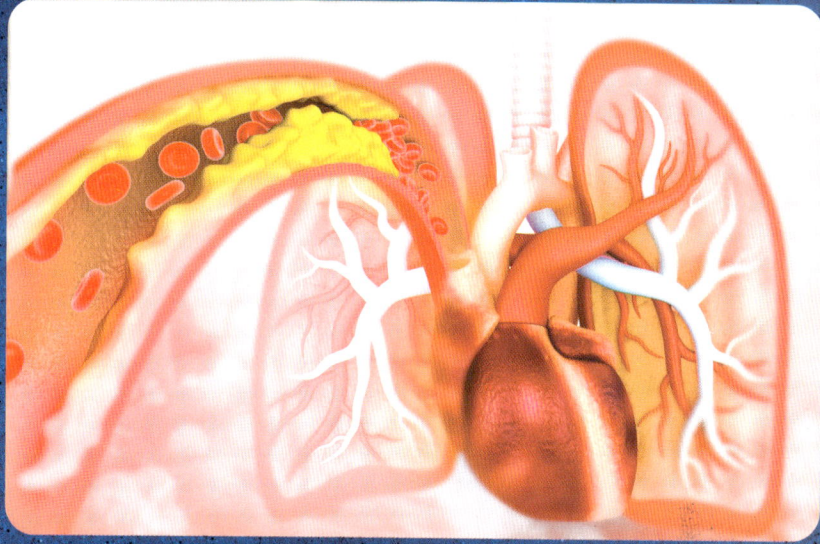

One of the most well known of these is coronary heart disease, which is when the flow of blood to the heart is blocked. This blockage is often caused by fatty deposits building up in the arteries and making them narrower – a condition called atherosclerosis. The condition also comes with an increased risk of blood clots. Your risk of developing atherosclerosis and coronary heart disease is higher if you have high blood pressure, high cholesterol or diabetes. Both atherosclerosis and coronary heart disease can also cause an irregular heartbeat called atrial fibrillation (AF), the signs of which include heart palpitations, feeling dizzy and chest pain. While having high blood pressure doesn't directly cause AF, it does contribute to both atherosclerosis and coronary heart disease, which can both cause AF. AF raises the risk of having a stroke (more on stroke risk later on).

Much like hypertension, coronary heart disease doesn't always have any noticeable symptoms, especially at first, but there are some as the condition develops. The most common is pain in the chest, also known as angina. The angina, in itself, is not life threatening, but it is a warning sign that something's not right. Other symptoms include feeling breathless, having pain in the neck, shoulders, jaw or arms, feeling dizzy and faint, or feeling sick. Coronary heart disease is usually diagnosed after assessing your likely risk, followed by scans and X-rays to see how the heart is functioning. Once you have coronary heart disease it cannot be cured, but there are treatment options that can lower the risk of it leading to a heart attack.

A heart attack happens when the flow of blood to the heart is blocked, usually by a blood clot. This clot can be caused by a fatty deposit in the arteries rupturing. It is very serious, and emergency medical help should be sought immediately. The main symptoms include a heavy, tight pain in the chest; pain in other parts of the body, including your left arm or both arms, jaw, neck, back and stomach; feeling very lightheaded; sweating; feeling breathless or wheezing; feeling or being sick; and feeling very anxious or panicked. Recovering from a heart attack can take time and it will be important to reduce your risk of another heart attack going forwards, which means improving your fitness, introducing lifestyle changes, and the right medication. There are serious complications that can occur during a heart attack, which are life-threatening, including cardiogenic shock and a heart rupture.

Another serious complication of coronary heart disease is heart failure, which is when the heart becomes stiff and weak, meaning that it can't pump blood around the body properly. It's a long-term condition that gets worse over time, and it cannot be cured. There are, however, treatments to manage the symptoms, ranging from lifestyle interventions to medicine and surgery. High blood pressure is a significant risk factor when it comes to heart failure, as having high blood pressure for a long time can put extra strain on the heart until it fails.

STROKE RISK
One in four people over 25 will experience a stroke in their lifetime.[2]

31

UNDERSTANDING HYPERTENSION

OTHER TYPES OF CVD

Arterial thrombosis is the term used to describe a blood clot that forms in an artery. As we've mentioned, a heart attack is often caused by a blood clot blocking the blood flow into the heart, but arterial thrombosis can cause blockages in other parts of the body too. This can cause damage to the brain, heart, kidneys or eyes, as well as issues with limbs.

The different types of CVD are caused by these blockages in other parts of the body. Along with heart attacks, the other major cause for concern is having a stroke. A stroke is caused when blood flow to the brain is blocked, which is a very serious condition that can be life threatening. If a person survives the stroke, it can leave lasting brain damage, impacting speech and movement, and the recovery can be slow.

Symptoms can come on very quickly and are usually characterised by a drooping or weakness in one side of the face, weakness or numbness in one or both arms, and problems with speech, such as slurring. These signs of a stroke and the need to get help are summarised in the acronym FAST, which stands for Face, Arms, Speech and Time to call the emergency medical service in your country.

Strokes can happen at any age, though they are more likely as you age. The most common type of stroke is an ischaemic stroke, which is when a blood clot blocks the blood flow to the brain. There is also a haemorrhagic stroke, which is caused by a burst blood vessel. Some people have what's called a transient ischaemic attack, otherwise known as a TIA or 'mini stroke'. In these cases, the symptoms of the stroke last for less than 24 hours and the blood flow to the brain is only temporarily disrupted. Urgent medical attention is still required, though, as a TIA can mean you're at risk of a full stroke. Other risk factors for a stroke include age (being over 50), ethnicity (being from a Black or South Asian background) and an unhealthy lifestyle. Hypertension increases the risk of a stroke, as does high cholesterol and diabetes.

If there is a blockage in the blood vessels leading to the limbs, this can cause peripheral arterial disease (PAD). This can cause numbness or weakness in your legs, muscle wastage in the legs, or ulcers on the feet and legs that don't heal. This condition can develop slowly over time, but once diagnosed it can be treated with lifestyle changes, as well as medication to treat the underlying causes. The main causes are smoking, diabetes, hypertension and high cholesterol.

CVD also includes aortic disease, which is an umbrella term

KIDNEY PROBLEMS
Long-term high blood pressure can seriously affect your kidney function

Kidneys play an important role in your body. Most people have two kidneys, which filter the blood and remove waste products from the body. They also help to balance the pH level of the blood, produce glucose, make a protein that increases blood pressure, and produce certain hormones. The adrenal glands sit on top of the kidneys, which are responsible for producing cortisol, which helps to manage stress, maintain blood pressure and support immune function. If you have hypertension, this can impact the blood vessels that lead in and out of the kidneys, making them weaker and less flexible. This means that the blood flow to the kidneys can be reduced, making it harder for them to do their job and even leading to scarring on the delicate tissue in the kidneys. If the kidneys are damaged, they cannot regulate blood pressure. Over time, this can lead to kidney disease, and if untreated, kidney failure.

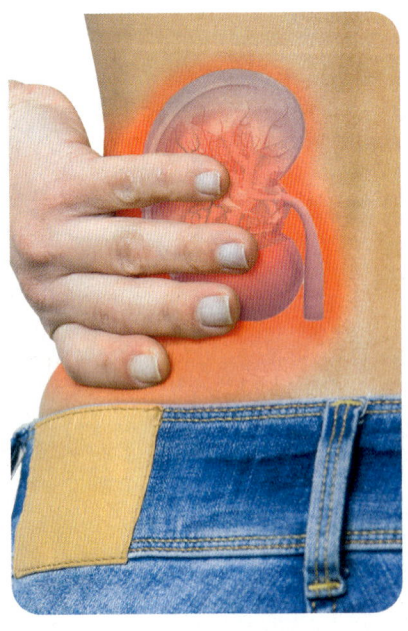

RISKS AND HEALTH IMPLICATIONS

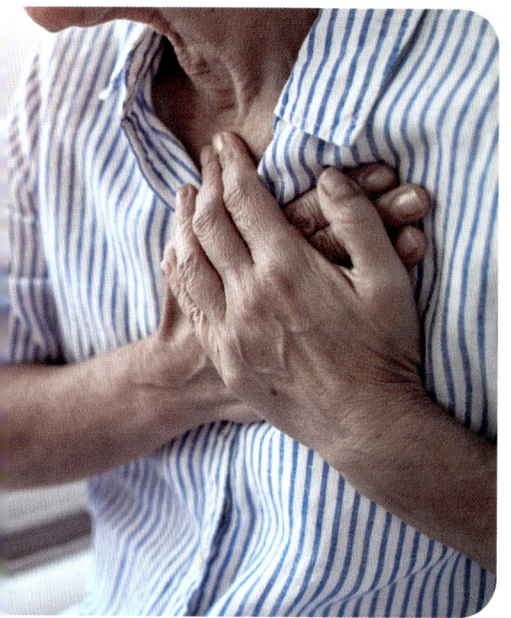

> ### EYE PROBLEMS
> High blood pressure can impact on your eye health
>
> When you go for a check-up on your eyes, you may be asked whether you have been diagnosed with high blood pressure. This is due to the known link between eye health and hypertension. In fact, an optometrist can even be the first person to spot the signs of high blood pressure when looking at the eyes, as the blood vessels in the retinas can become narrower and less flexible as a result. High blood pressure can lead to a condition called hypertensive retinopathy, which is when the blood vessels in the eye become damaged to the point where they impact vision. Early symptoms include blurred vision and headaches. More serious cases can even lead to vision loss or bleeding. It's important to seek help if you notice blurred vision so that an examination can be carried out to see if hypertensive retinopathy is the cause. The treatment is to get the hypertension under control through medication or lifestyle changes.

for conditions that affect the largest blood vessel, the aorta. This includes an aortic aneurysm, which is a swelling in the blood vessel that carries blood from the heart to the stomach. They may not cause any issues, but there's a risk that they can burst, which is a far more serious condition. Treatment for an aortic aneurysm includes using medicines that lower your blood pressure to prevent the aneurysm from getting worse. If the aortic aneurysm gets bigger, it could be that it needs to be surgically removed.

Most CVDs are actually preventable and are linked to unhealthy lifestyle factors or environmental factors. This includes things like smoking, drinking alcohol, eating an unhealthy diet, being overweight, being physically inactive and air pollution. Someone with hypertension is at more risk of developing CVDs and heart problems, which is why monitoring blood pressure is so important. The earlier that these warning signs are caught, the easier it is to prevent them developing further into one of these more serious conditions.

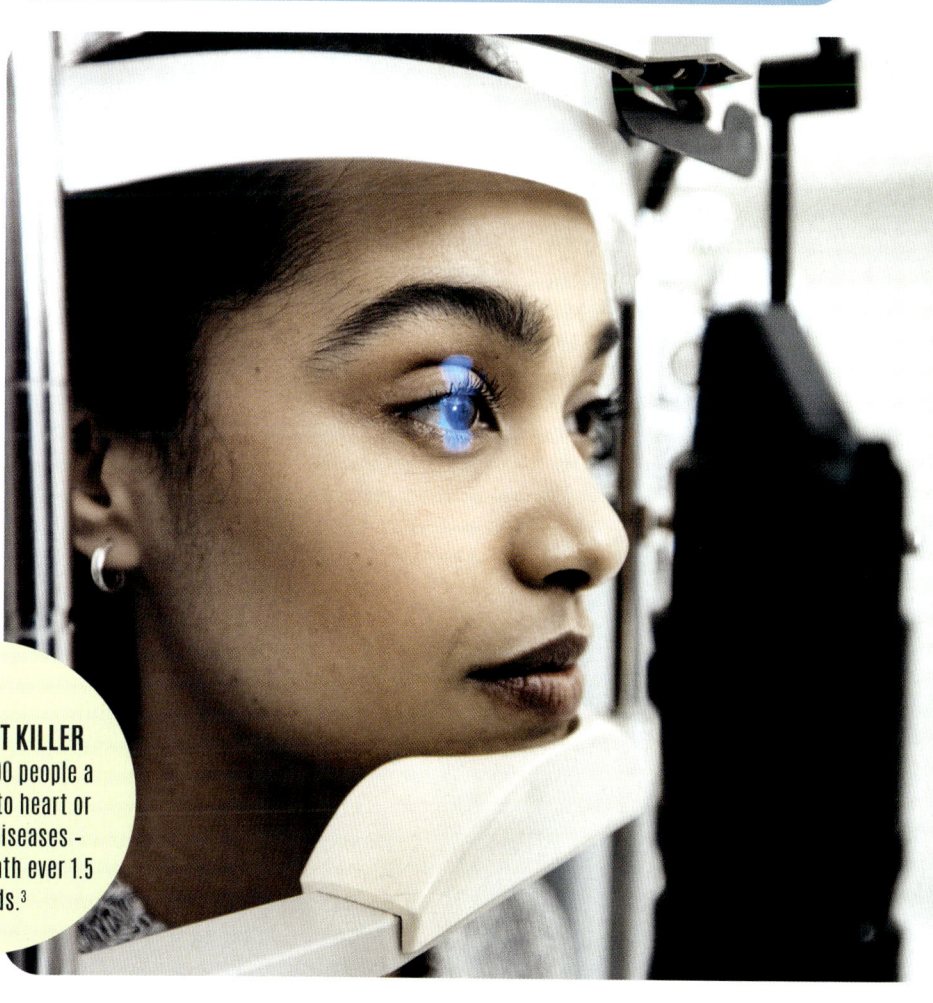

THE BIGGEST KILLER
In 2021, 55,000 people a day died due to heart or circulatory diseases - that's one death ever 1.5 seconds.[3]

33

UNDERSTANDING
HYPERTENSION

VASCULAR DEMENTIA

Reduced blood flow is also the cause of vascular dementia, and having hypertension means that you're more at risk. Vascular dementia is when there is reduced blood flow to the brain, causing gradual but permanent damage to the brain cells. Symptoms include having slow thoughts, finding it hard to concentrate, feeling confused, changes to mood and/or personality, difficulty understanding, and having trouble walking or balancing. As the condition progresses over the months and years, a person may eventually need round-the-clock support if they're unable to cope with everyday activities.

If vascular dementia is caught early, there are treatments that may be able to stop or slow down its progression. It's most common in people aged over 65, and there are various tests that help to determine a diagnosis, including assessments of symptoms and mental ability, a full medical history and a brain scan.

The main cause of vascular dementia is the sustained reduced blood flow to the brain. This can be due to things like a stroke or multiple TIAs, causing irreversible damage to the brain, as well as the narrowing of blood vessels. The underlying causes can vary, but hypertension and diabetes are both significant contributors. The damaged brain cells cannot be treated or restored, however by tackling the underlying causes, it can be possible to limit further damage. This can include eating a healthy diet and reaching and/or maintaining a healthy weight; giving up smoking and cutting down on alcohol; and building physical fitness. Medicines can also treat the underlying hypertension or high cholesterol, and reduce the chance of blood clots. However, vascular dementia will continue to progress over time and symptoms will worsen – though it's impossible to predict the speed at which this will happen. Some people with vascular dementia also have Alzheimer's disease, which is caused by a build-up of certain proteins in the brain. These proteins can seriously impact memory, in particular recent memory. When a person has more than one kind of dementia, this is known as 'mixed dementia'.

As you can see, there are some very serious complications that can result from having high blood pressure. Reducing your blood pressure, even by a little, can start to bring down your risk of these health problems. Many of the complications we've talked about here have similar underlying causes and similar risk factors. But they also have similar treatments and interventions. Therefore, the steps you take to get your blood pressure under control will also help to prevent and lower your risk of these more serious and life-changing conditions.

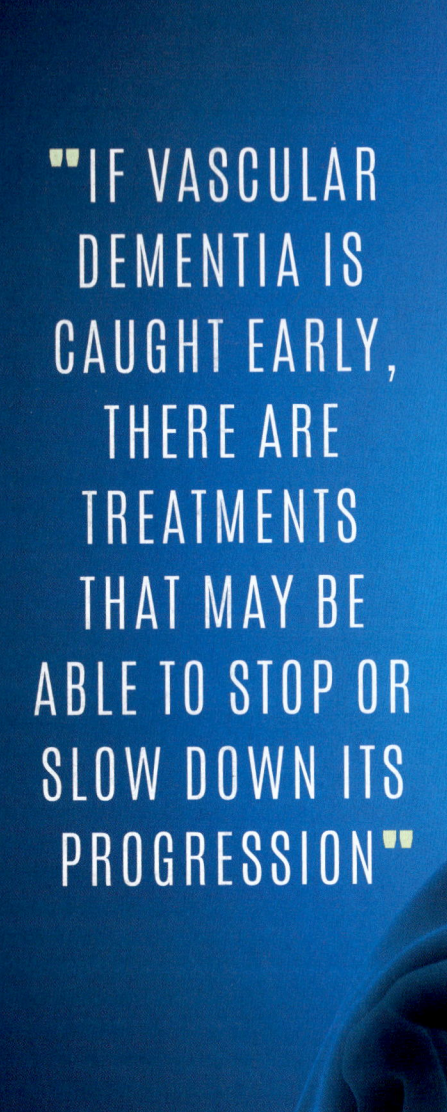

"IF VASCULAR DEMENTIA IS CAUGHT EARLY, THERE ARE TREATMENTS THAT MAY BE ABLE TO STOP OR SLOW DOWN ITS PROGRESSION"

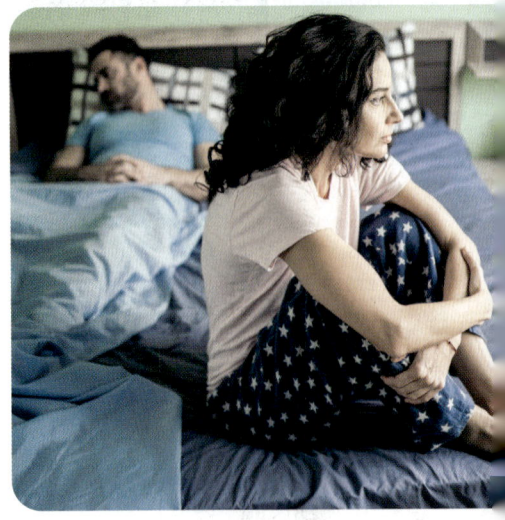

RISKS AND HEALTH IMPLICATIONS

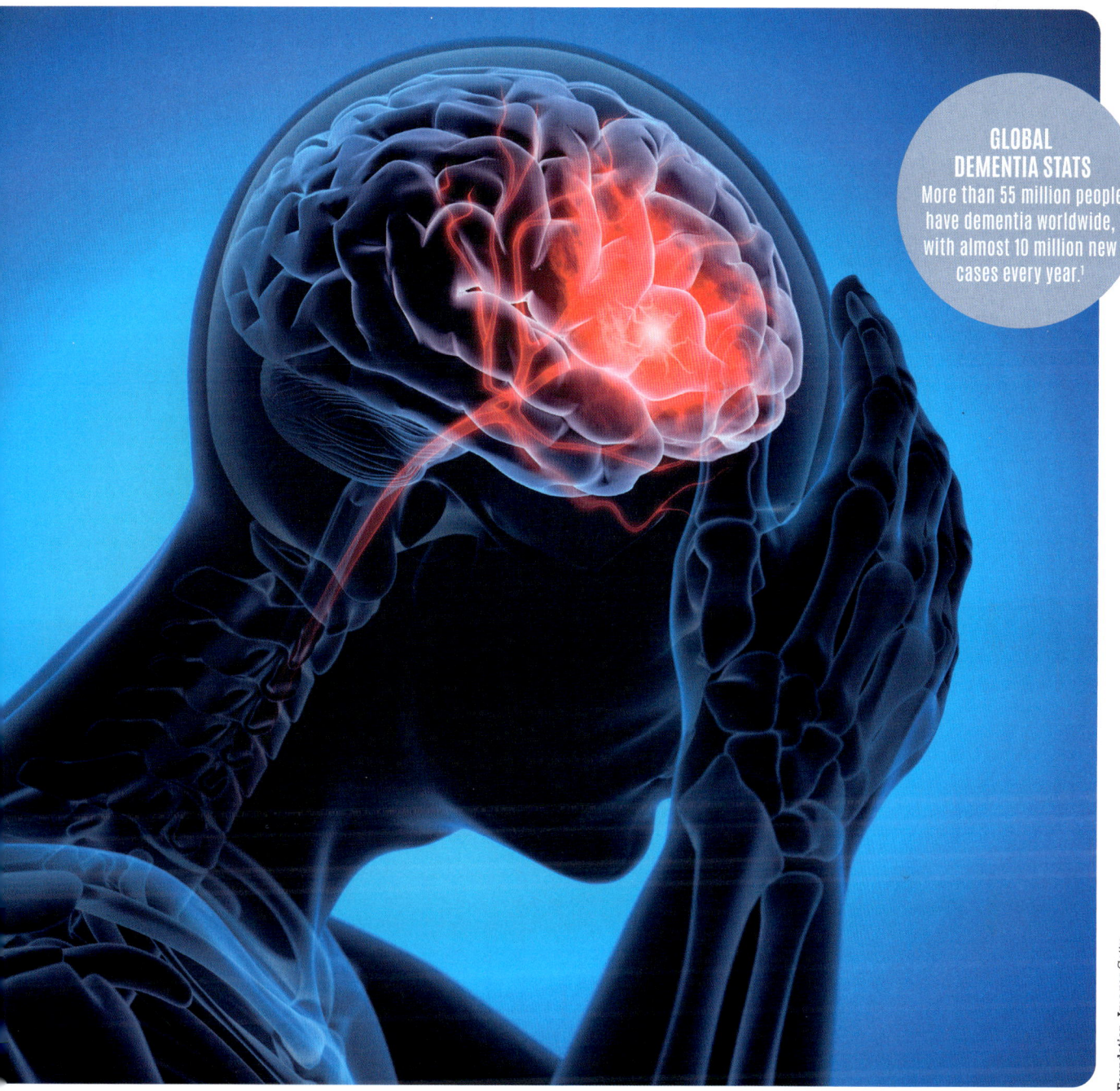

GLOBAL DEMENTIA STATS
More than 55 million people have dementia worldwide, with almost 10 million new cases every year.[1]

SEXUAL CONDITIONS

Hypertension can have some effect on sexual function in both men and women

Having high blood pressure can cause some loss of sexual function. In men, this can mean erectile dysfunction, due to the blood vessels leading to the penis being damaged or narrowed, preventing normal blood flow to the area.

Alongside hypertension, other causes of erectile dysfunction include diabetes, smoking and drinking a lot of alcohol. Lifestyle changes or medications to lower blood pressure can help to improve sexual function. In women, high blood pressure can reduce the blood flow to the vagina, resulting in reduced arousal and sex drive, and an increase of vaginal dryness. Again, treating the underlying cause of hypertension can improve the symptoms.

UNDERSTANDING
HYPERTENSION

GETTING A DIAGNOSIS

UNDIAGNOSED HYPERTENSION
This is a big risk factor for stroke, heart attacks and dementia if left untreated for a long time.

What happens from your first high blood pressure reading to a hypertension diagnosis

Many people don't know that they have high blood pressure when they are diagnosed, as there are few signs or symptoms. This means that it can come as a shock and cause a lot of worry. You won't be diagnosed with high blood pressure from a single high reading – blood pressure naturally fluctuates throughout the day and can be impacted by normal daily activity. But it is a warning sign that there needs to be further checks and investigations.

If you have your blood pressure taken as part of a routine health check-up and the reading is showing as higher than it should be, this will be noted on your medical records. If it's in the pre-hypertension stage, then there may not be a need for further checks. The practitioner may instead give advice on lifestyle interventions that can stop it progressing and check again in six months or a year. However, if the reading is very high, then you will usually be referred for further tests. If you have taken your own reading at home with a blood pressure machine and you find that you have high numbers, you should call your doctor and make an appointment for a check-up to confirm your readings and see if any further tests are needed. Readings at home are not always as accurate as ones taken in a clinic, which is why the threshold for high blood pressure and the different stages of hypertension are lower than readings taken in a clinical setting.

Further checks and tests

If you are referred to a doctor or specialist after a high blood pressure reading, you will usually be seen in person to do more tests. The doctor will normally retake the blood pressure readings. Ideally you would be checked when you're feeling calm and relaxed. The doctor should then take a reading in both arms, just in case there is a significant difference between them. The doctor may need to repeat the readings if there is a difference between them, and if there is still a difference, then the arm with the higher blood pressure reading is normally used going forwards. If the readings are high, then the doctor may repeat the readings just to double check.

Sometimes a doctor will use an automated blood pressure machine with a digital display of your numbers. However, they may also take a manual reading. In this case the cuff is attached to an inflation bulb with an analogue pressure gauge. The doctor can then listen to your blood flow using a stethoscope to determine your blood pressure numbers. Sometimes this is a matter of preference, but there are times when it's better to use a manual

GETTING A DIAGNOSIS

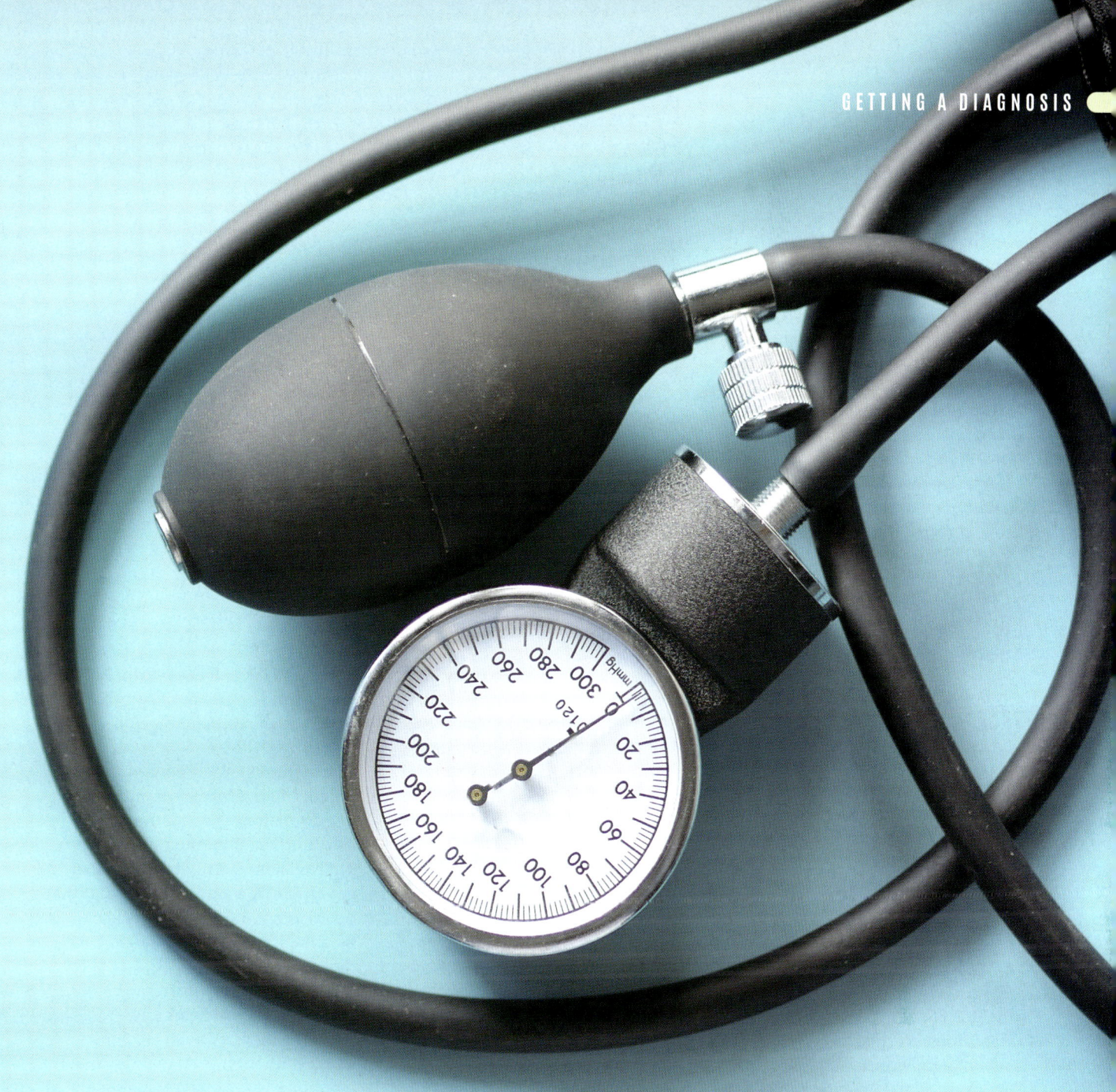

method. For example, in a person with an irregular pulse, an automated device may not always give an accurate reading.

If your blood pressure readings fall within the Stage 1 or Stage 2 hypertension levels, up to about 180/120 mmHG, then you will usually have to undergo further tests to measure your blood pressure over a period of time. There are two main ways that this is done.

The first is to do something called 'ambulatory blood pressure monitoring' or ABPM. This is a

"READINGS AT HOME ARE NOT ALWAYS AS ACCURATE AS ONES TAKEN IN A CLINIC"

24-hour test to see how your blood pressure changes throughout a full day as you go about your normal activity. It is a cuff worn on the arm connected to a reading device attached to a belt or strap. Blood pressure is then monitored at regular intervals – usually at least twice an hour – which enables an average blood pressure reading to be calculated. The cuff and device can't get wet, so that means no baths or showers, but you can do most normal day-to-day activities. You need to be up and moving about for this test to be effective,

Image Getty

37

UNDERSTANDING HYPERTENSION

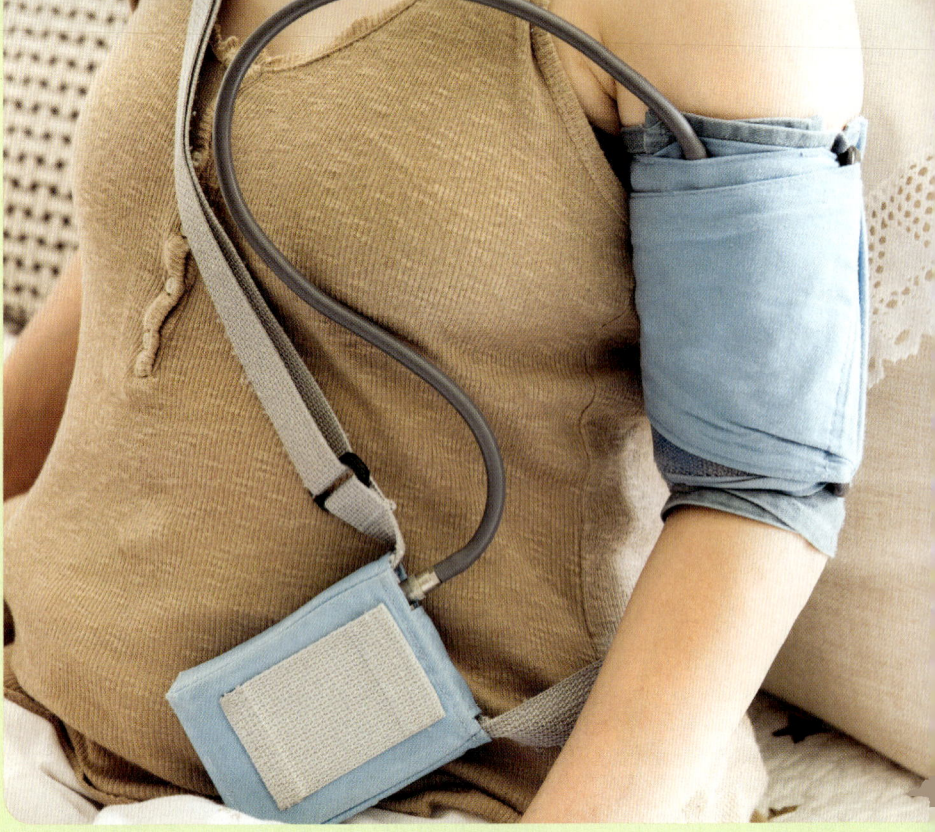

so it may not be suitable for those with mobility issues or those with other health problems that limit their movement.

The other option is home blood pressure monitoring (HBPM), which uses an at-home blood pressure monitor. You may be given one to take home for the duration of the testing period. You will also be shown how to use it to get the most accurate readings. The doctor will tell you how often to test your blood pressure and for how long – usually for up to a week. Again, this means that an average blood pressure reading can be taken. Using this average data along with the in-clinic readings, the doctor can then confirm a diagnosis of hypertension and the stage.

Building the full picture

If the initial in-clinic blood pressure readings are much higher, above 180/120 mmHG, the doctor will likely ask about other symptoms to check for things like chest pain, signs of heart failure or signs of problems with the kidneys, which could need immediate and urgent treatment. They will usually want to follow up with further readings and tests to determine if there is an underlying cause for the high blood pressure. In the case of people under 40, doctors will be looking for a potential cause of secondary hypertension.

As well as the blood pressure readings, the doctor will want to build up a full picture of your overall health. This will mean asking about your activity levels, your diet, whether you smoke and whether you drink alcohol. They will also ask questions about your family history regarding hypertension, strokes and heart disease. All this information will help to determine your individual risk of developing serious health problems to inform the right treatment plan.

According to NICE guidelines in the UK, a diagnosis of hypertension is confirmed in people with an in-clinic blood pressure reading of 140/90 mmHG or higher and an ABPM or HBPM average of 135/85 mmHG or higher. The diagnosis is then broken down into Stage 1, Stage 2 or Stage 3 (which is severe), depending on the in-clinic readings in conjunction with the ABPM or HBPM.

Sometimes other tests might be needed to confirm a diagnosis of hypertension, to see if there is anything else potentially causing it. This is especially true if you're not typically a person who would be at risk of high blood pressure (ie a healthy weight, balanced diet, regularly active etc). This might include, for example, a blood test to check for any irregularities, a cholesterol test, kidney function tests and thyroid function tests. Some people may also have checks on their heart, including an electrocardiogram to look at the heart function. It's important to rule out any other health problems before starting on a treatment plan.

Getting a diagnosis of hypertension means that you can start to look at treatment options, which is usually a combination of lifestyle factors and medication, depending on the severity of the hypertension. It also means that you will be checked more often, and you may have to have blood pressure readings a lot more frequently. This is to ensure that your treatment plan is working and to check that your readings are not continuing to go upwards.

"AS WELL AS THE BLOOD PRESSURE READINGS, THE DOCTOR WILL WANT TO BUILD UP A FULL PICTURE OF YOUR OVERALL HEALTH"

UNUSUAL BLOOD PRESSURE READINGS

There are some cases when you might get different readings in different situations

In some people, readings can be quite different between those taken in a clinical setting and those taken at home. One reason for this is 'white coat syndrome' or 'white coat effect', which refers to those who have higher than normal blood pressure readings in a clinical setting, but not when at home. This is due to people feeling nervous or stressed when in a clinic and around medical professionals, causing a temporary rise in blood pressure. If it happens regularly, you may be advised to try taking readings at home to get a clearer picture of your health. You can also discuss ways to make the experience less stressful with your clinician to help get a better idea of your normal blood pressure.

This is something that can happen to people both with and without hypertension. If someone has blood pressure readings over the threshold for hypertension in the clinic, but is lower than the threshold at home, this is sometimes called 'white coat hypertension'. If it happens the other way around – ie the readings are normal in the clinic but routinely elevated at home – then this is sometimes called 'masked hypertension'.

SEEK SUPPORT
If you are diagnosed with hypertension, ask your doctor if there are any support groups you could go to for advice.

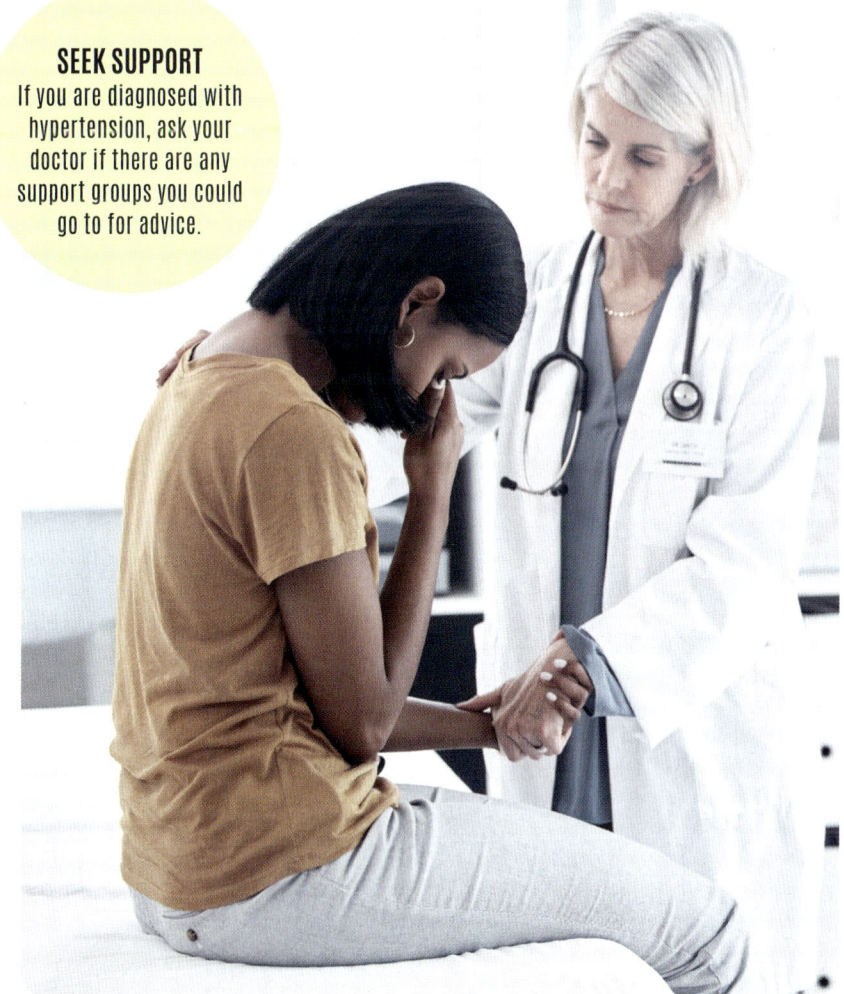

GETTING A DIAGNOSIS

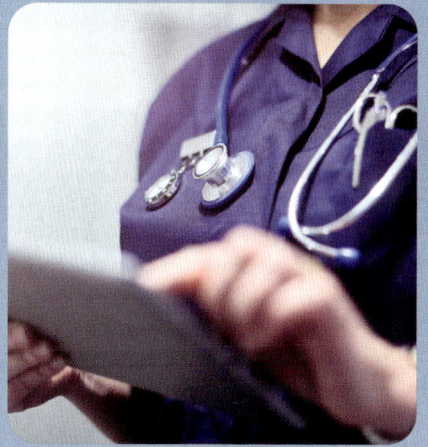

KNOW YOUR HISTORY

Before an appointment to talk about high blood pressure, get organised with what a doctor needs to know

When you are asked to go to an appointment to potentially be diagnosed with high blood pressure, you can make it easier by being prepared as much as possible for what they are going to ask you. The first thing you should be prepared for is questions about your current health, so think about how often you have a drink or do exercise – be honest, as this can help with your diagnosis and treatment plan. You should also ensure that you know your family history, as the doctor will need to ask questions about this. Has anyone in your family had heart disease and at what age? Has anyone in your family had a stroke and at what age? Is there type 2 diabetes in your family? Or vascular dementia? Is hypertension common in your family? You'll also be asked about other symptoms you might be experiencing, as well as any current medication you're taking. Don't forget to make a list of any regular supplements you might be taking, too.

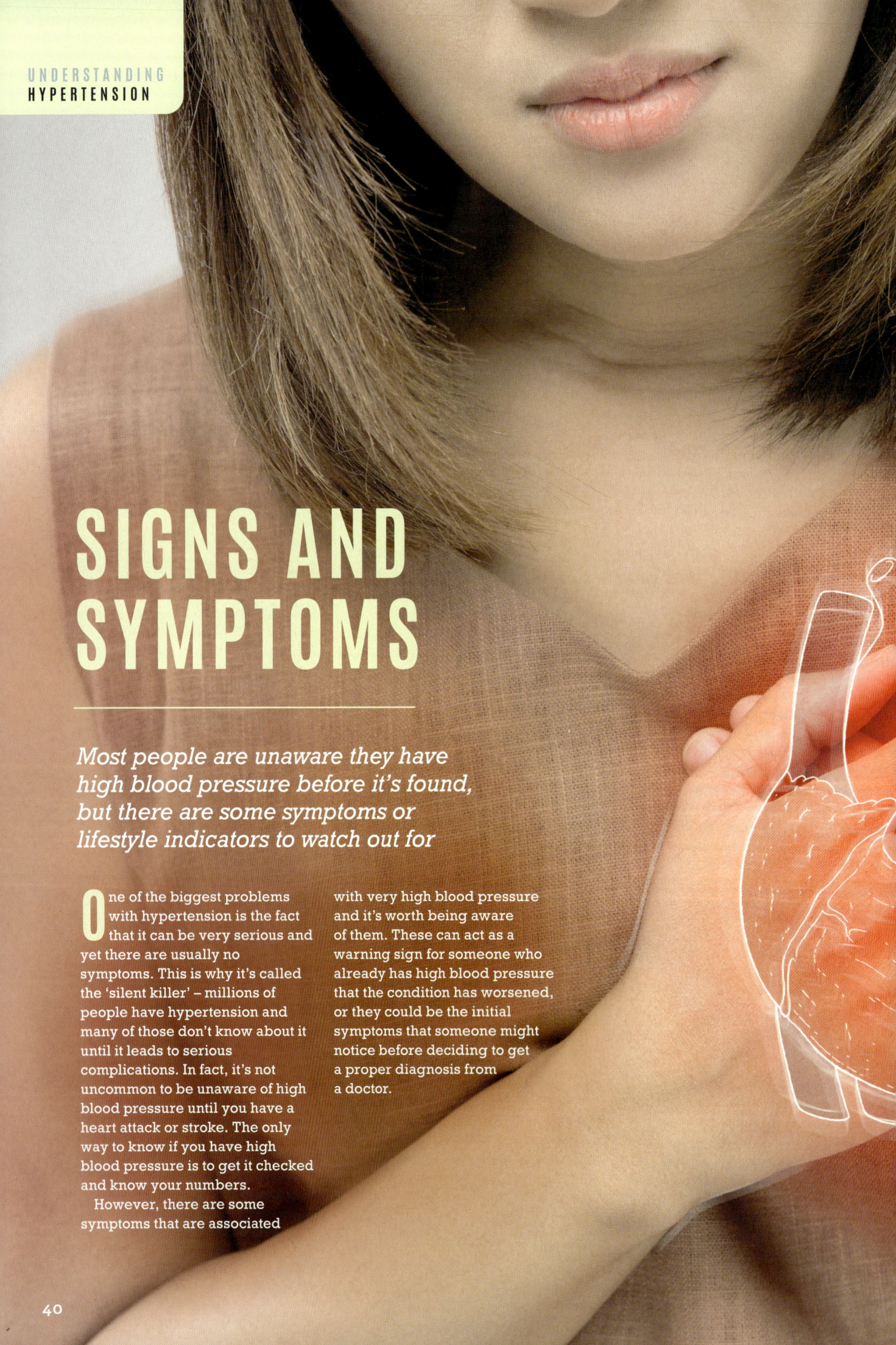

UNDERSTANDING
HYPERTENSION

SIGNS AND SYMPTOMS

Most people are unaware they have high blood pressure before it's found, but there are some symptoms or lifestyle indicators to watch out for

One of the biggest problems with hypertension is the fact that it can be very serious and yet there are usually no symptoms. This is why it's called the 'silent killer' – millions of people have hypertension and many of those don't know about it until it leads to serious complications. In fact, it's not uncommon to be unaware of high blood pressure until you have a heart attack or stroke. The only way to know if you have high blood pressure is to get it checked and know your numbers.

However, there are some symptoms that are associated with very high blood pressure and it's worth being aware of them. These can act as a warning sign for someone who already has high blood pressure that the condition has worsened, or they could be the initial symptoms that someone might notice before deciding to get a proper diagnosis from a doctor.

SIGNS AND SYMPTOMS

SYMPTOMS OF VERY HIGH BLOOD PRESSURE

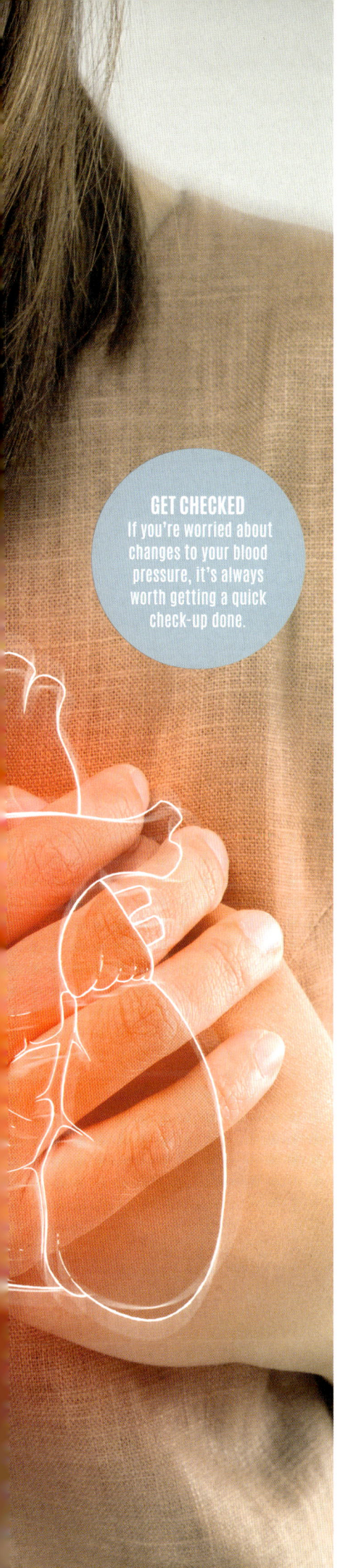

GET CHECKED
If you're worried about changes to your blood pressure, it's always worth getting a quick check-up done.

People with very severe hypertension – defined as being 180/120mmHG or higher, which is Stage 3 hypertension – may experience several different symptoms. If someone has any of these symptoms along with high blood pressure, this is a medical emergency and needs urgent referral. If you already have high blood pressure, be vigilant and keep up with your regular checks to ensure that your blood pressure is under control, but also be aware of the signs that things could be getting worse. Sometimes elevated blood pressure that is above this threshold is called a hypertensive crisis or a hypertensive emergency.

Severe hypertension can cause headaches due to the increased pressure around the brain. This is usually felt on both sides of the head. Some people experience chest pain and dizziness, particularly if your blood pressure elevates very suddenly. Some people also report finding it hard to breathe or feeling anxious and confused. Blurred vision can also be associated with high blood pressure, as can nosebleeds, nausea or vomiting. You may also experience an abnormal heart rhythm or a buzzing in the ears.

These symptoms are normally a sign that high blood pressure is causing a complication or serious problem, rather than being 'just' high blood pressure on its own. This is why it's essential to get immediate help. There are some symptoms that should never be ignored, particularly if you already know you have hypertension. The quicker you can get medical treatment the better.

You should speak to a medical professional if you find that you are having more regular headaches than normal, or if you are having blurred vision. You should also get a check-up if you are experiencing chest pain that comes and goes. If you have any other unusual symptoms and you're already diagnosed with hypertension, then it's better to be safe and seen than it is to ignore it.

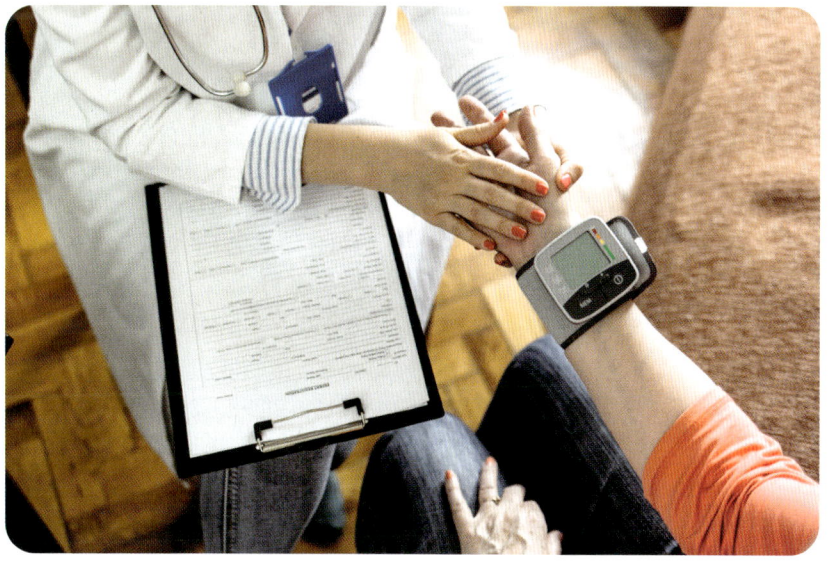

Images Getty

41

UNDERSTANDING HYPERTENSION

SIGNS OF HEALTH PROBLEMS ASSOCIATED WITH HYPERTENSION

As hypertension usually has no symptoms on its own, it's often the signs and symptoms of health complications and issues that are caused by sustained high blood pressure that can prompt people to see a doctor in the first place.

If you have any symptoms like occasional chest pain, regular shortness of breath, pain in your neck, arms, jaw or shoulders, or feel faint and nauseous often, this should trigger a check-up. This can be a sign that you have developed coronary heart disease, which could be because you have undiagnosed or uncontrolled hypertension. See the box below for the signs of a heart attack, as these are similar but are often sudden onset and more severe. Also watch out for the signs of heart failure, which can develop slowly over time or very quickly. The symptoms of heart failure can be similar to other health conditions, so if you experience any of these, especially if you have a hypertension diagnosis already, then you need to speak to your doctor. Breathlessness after an activity or even at rest is one sign, as is feeling tired a lot of the time and especially after exercise. You may also feel lightheaded or frequently faint. Some people also feel dizzy or have swollen legs and ankles, a fast heart rate or a persistent cough. These can all be signs that the heart is struggling to pump blood around the body.

You should be aware of the symptoms of a stroke, as this is another problem that can be caused by high blood pressure and again can be the first time that someone becomes aware of having hypertension. We've covered the key symptoms in our feature on the risks and health implications of hypertension (pages 30-35), including face weakness, arm weakness and speech problems. Other symptoms that you should watch out for include numbness or weakness down one side of the body, blurred vision or loss of sight in one or both eyes, finding it hard to think of words, feeling confused or suffering memory loss, feeling dizzy, losing balance or having a severe headache.

WHEN TO GET EMERGENCY HELP
Know what a heart attack looks like and get medical support immediately

One of the biggest concerns with uncontrolled hypertension is a heart attack, so you should be aware of the main symptoms and call emergency services straight away. You will need to get to a hospital as soon as possible to begin immediate treatment. The key signs of a heart attack are:

Chest pain
This is often described as a heavy pain, a feeling of pressure, squeezing or general tightness.

Other pain
You may experience pain in other parts of the body spreading from the chest to the left arm (or both arms), jaw, neck, back or stomach.

Dizziness
You may feel lightheaded and dizzy, and sometimes you may have a strong feeling of anxiety or panic.

Breathlessness
You may feel as though you are short of breath or be coughing and/or wheezing.

Other symptoms
You may experience sickness or nausea, or find that you're sweating a lot.

Call 999 (UK), 911 (USA) or your country's emergency services if you experience any of these symptoms.

> "SOMETHING TO WATCH OUT FOR ARE SIGNS OF KIDNEY DISEASE"

SIGNS AND SYMPTOMS

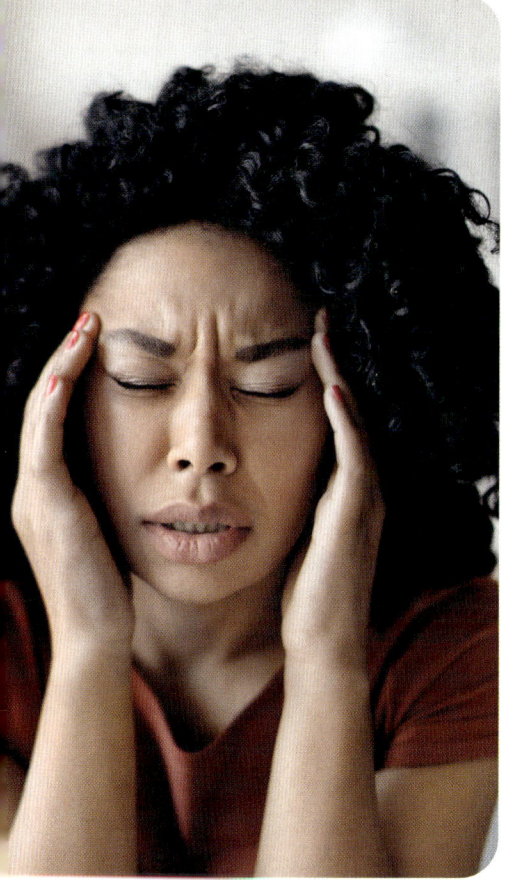

OTHER TYPES OF CHEST PAIN
If you have hypertension and are experiencing chest pain, there can be many underlying causes

You might be very worried if you know that you have high blood pressure and then start to get chest pain every now and then, as you instantly assume it's a problem with your heart. And while you should definitely get checked out as soon as possible (if it's severe and sudden, call emergency services), there are other reasons why you might get chest pain.

One of the most common explanations is heartburn or indigestion, which can cause a burning pain in the middle of your chest. Chest pain can also be a sign of an underlying chest infection, where chest pain is accompanied with a chesty cough, wheezing, breathlessness, a high temperature, headaches, aching joints or tiredness. It's also possible to injure the muscles in your chest, which can be very painful, or you may experience inflammation in your rib cage. Some people also suffer chest pain when they're feeling anxious. It's important to visit your doctor to figure out the cause of your chest pain.

Sometimes these symptoms can pass quite quickly, which can make it seem like it's nothing serious, but you should still seek medical assistance quickly as it can lead to a bigger stroke if not treated or identified.

Something else to watch out for are the signs of kidney disease, especially if you have hypertension and particularly if it's at a higher stage. The main symptoms are tiredness; swollen hands, feet or ankles; being short of breath; feeling sick; and noticing blood in your urine. Other symptoms can be easily dismissed as something else, such as weight loss, loss of appetite, insomnia, itchy skin or muscle cramps. If you have any of these signs, you should speak to your doctor as it's important to get the right treatment started as soon as possible.

BETTER SAFE THAN SORRY
Always speak up if you're concerned about a symptom - it's never a waste of time.

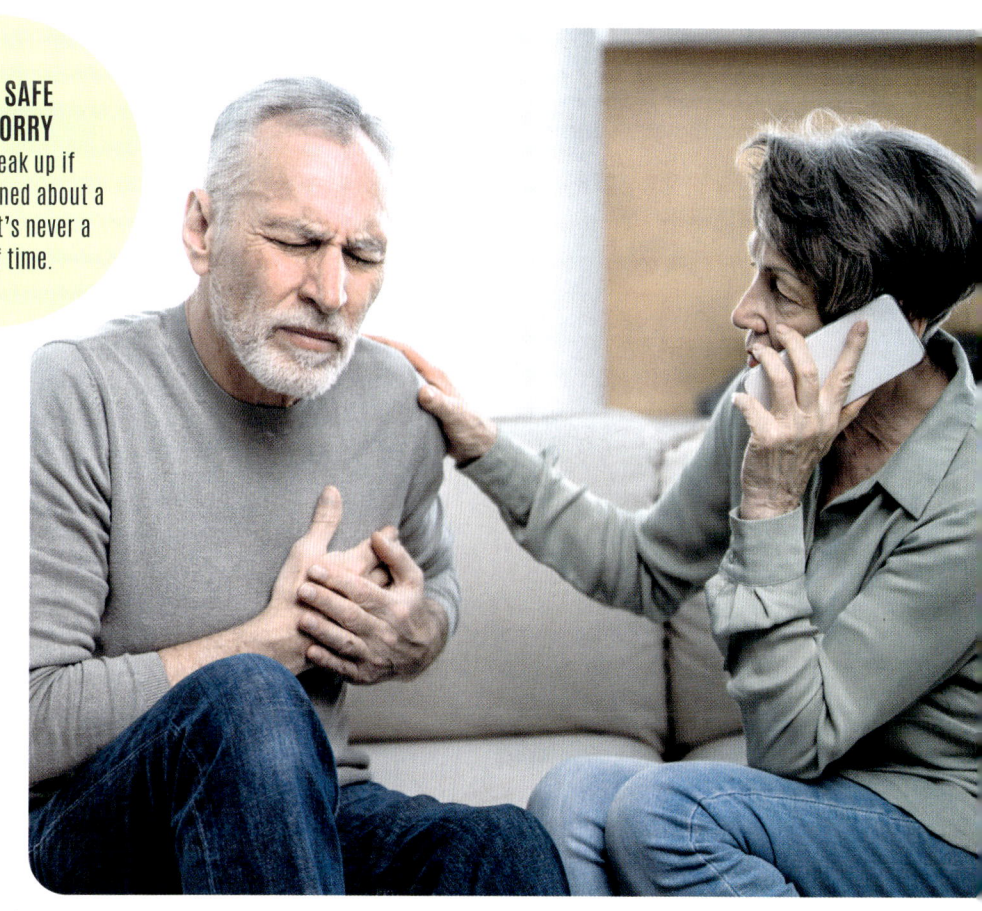

Images Getty

UNDERSTANDING HYPERTENSION

LIFESTYLE INDICATORS OF HIGH BLOOD PRESSURE

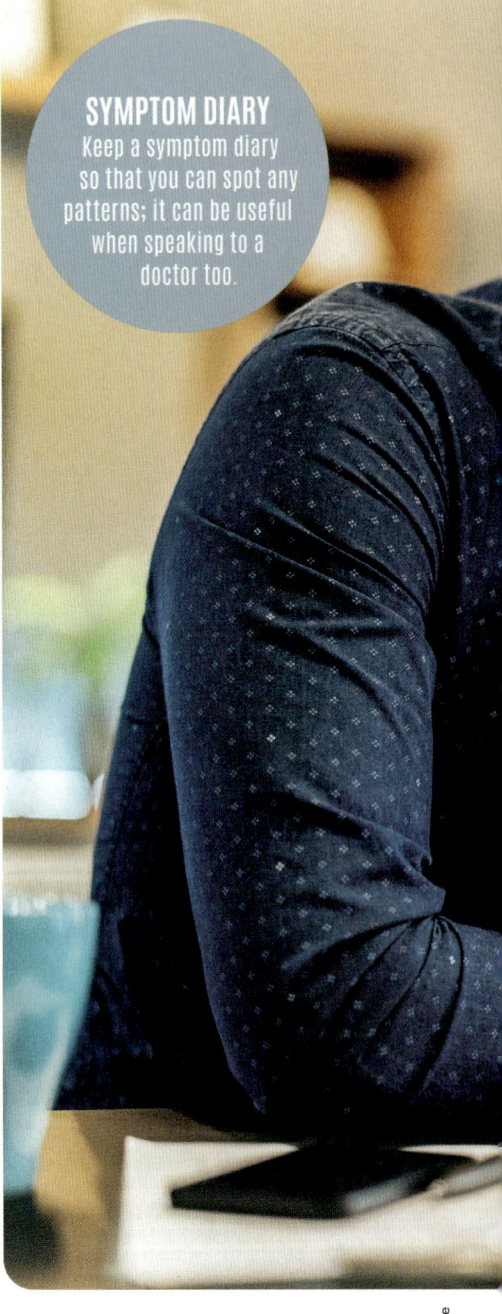

SYMPTOM DIARY
Keep a symptom diary so that you can spot any patterns; it can be useful when speaking to a doctor too.

With such limited symptoms to watch out for to indicate that you might have high blood pressure, you should also be looking to your lifestyle to see if there are any signs of potential hypertension. As you're aware, there are certain risk factors that make it more likely that a person can develop hypertension. It is therefore a good idea to take audit of certain lifestyle traits and, if you meet any of these criteria, you should definitely get your blood pressure checked as soon as you can. If you already have hypertension, then these are the areas you will need to focus on to help bring your blood pressure down.

Your weight is always a good indicator of whether you might be likely to have hypertension. We know that having excess weight is a significant risk factor, but what are you looking for? Obesity, in particular, is known to come with a high chance that you will also have high blood pressure – in fact, in the USA, 40% of the obese population also have hypertension.[1] Obesity is often defined by the BMI metric; those with a BMI of over 30 are considered obese, while those with a BMI of over 40 are considered severely obese. However, for those who have an Asian, Chinese, Middle Eastern, Black African or African-Caribbean family history, the threshold for obesity is a BMI of 27.5 or higher.

If you fall into this higher BMI category, or even if you are considered overweight rather than obese, it's a sign that you are more at risk of high blood pressure and therefore should get checked. Consider where your excess weight is distributed; if you carry more fat around your stomach, this can be another risk factor and another sign that you should get checked. We know that BMI is not a perfect measure, especially for those who carry a lot of muscle, but as a general number to monitor and to trigger a check-up, it can be useful.

Think about whether your lifestyle is healthy, too. If you smoke, then you should definitely take that as a sign to get your blood pressure checked, no matter how often you have a cigarette. Your risk of having hypertension is so much higher that you shouldn't leave it to chance. When it comes to alcohol, your risk rises the more you drink. If you find that you're drinking more than a couple of nights a week, and more than a couple of drinks at a time, it's worth getting your blood pressure checked out to see if there is any impact. Many people drink more than they realise and might not see it as a sign that they should be getting their blood pressure checked, however it's easy to creep in to the danger zone. If you're having a drink with dinner

> "YOUR WEIGHT IS ALWAYS A GOOD INDICATOR OF WHETHER YOU MIGHT BE LIKELY TO HAVE HYPERTENSION"

[1] The relationship between obesity and hypertension: an updated comprehensive overview on vicious twins, Hypertension Research, October 2017.

SIGNS AND SYMPTOMS

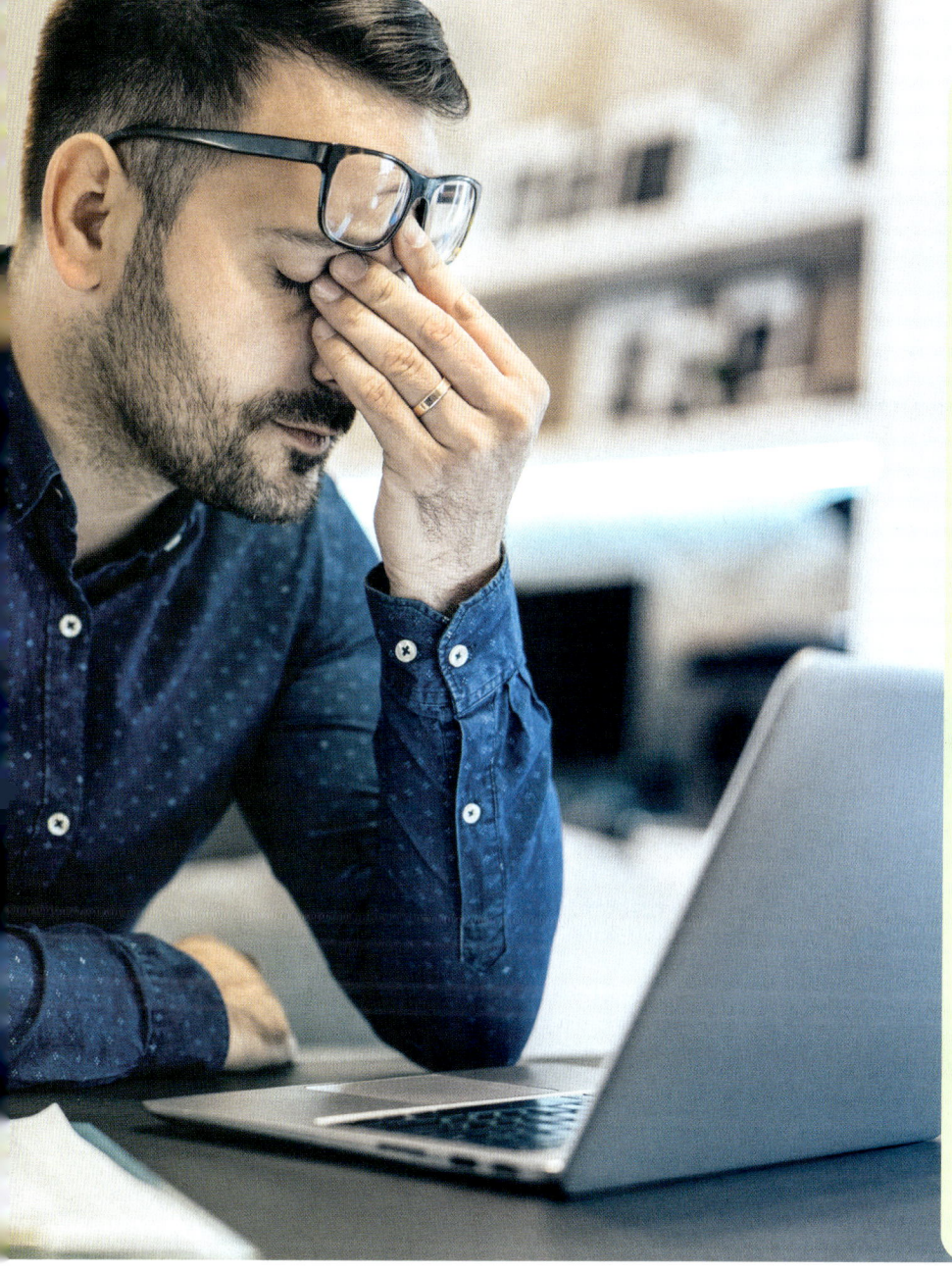

MENTAL HEALTH AND HYPERTENSION

How to spot the early signs of mental health conditions when diagnosed with high blood pressure

Being diagnosed with hypertension can affect your mental wellbeing. You may find it harder to make the lifestyle changes needed to help treat high blood pressure, and be more likely to do things that make your blood pressure worse. Signs of an anxiety disorder include feeling irritable, being worried, a feeling of dread, difficulty concentrating and insomnia. Symptoms of depression include hopelessness or sadness, a lack of energy, finding it hard to do things you usually enjoy, and a sense of agitation.

every night, for example, you could be easily exceeding the recommended weekly allowance, while also not giving your body a chance to recover.

Diet also plays a big part in how at risk you are. If you're worried that your diet could be contributing to poor health outcomes, get your blood pressure checked for peace of mind. This is especially true if you rely a lot on ultra-processed foods, ie foods that are packaged and convenient, usually with numerous ingredients you wouldn't find in a home kitchen. If you're prone to adding a lot of salt to your meals, or have a lot of salty meats, sauces or stocks, or takeaways, this is another warning sign to get checked.

The take-home message is that it's better to go for a check-up before you notice any serious symptoms. The symptoms of severe hypertension and the resulting health complications come at the point when it's already a problem. It's much better to be in tune with your body early on, either before you develop high blood pressure at all or when you've caught it at an early stage. If you feel like you are not eating well, not doing enough exercise, drinking or smoking too much, or not happy with your weight, take this as your sign to be proactive and get a quick, free blood pressure check. If you already have a diagnosis of hypertension, you should be even more vigilant for any indicators that your lifestyle could be impacting on your health.

Luckily, there is plenty that you can do to help treat high blood pressure, from lifestyle changes to medication, and the sooner you start, the more you can make a positive impact.

MANAGING HYPERTENSION

Discover how to get your blood pressure under control, whether that's via medication or making lifestyle changes

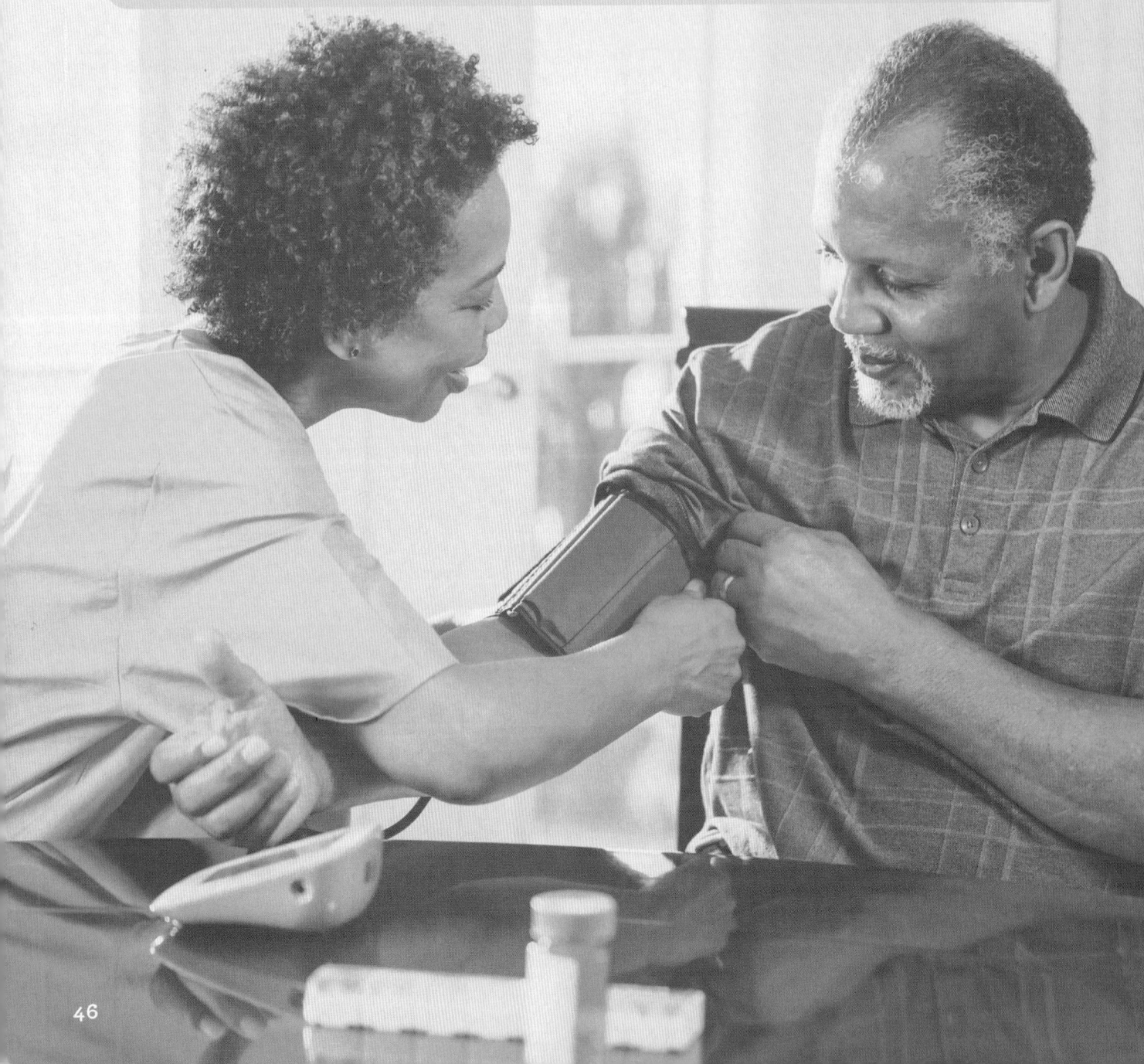

2

48
YOUR TREATMENT OPTIONS

52
MEDICATIONS FOR HYPERTENSION

56
WEIGHT MANAGEMENT

62
STRESS AND HYPERTENSION

66
MANAGING ALCOHOL CONSUMPTION

70
SMOKING AND HYPERTENSION

74
SUPPORT GROUPS AND RESOURCES

MANAGING HYPERTENSION

YOUR TREATMENT OPTIONS

You've been diagnosed with high blood pressure – what happens next? We give you an overview of the possible treatment options

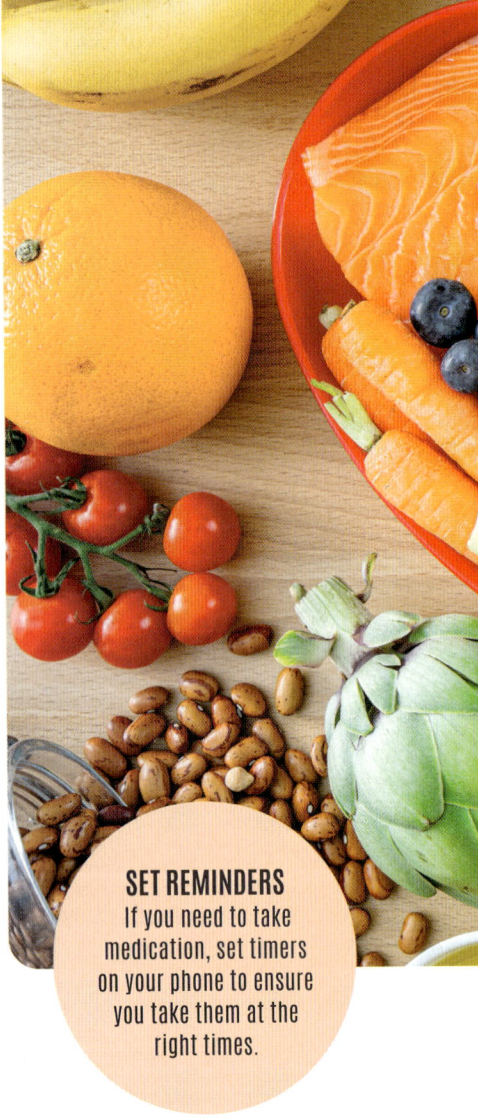

SET REMINDERS
If you need to take medication, set timers on your phone to ensure you take them at the right times.

Treating high blood pressure doesn't have one solution that fits all. Many factors are taken into consideration when it comes to creating a treatment plan. It depends on how high your blood pressure is (whether it's pre-hypertension or stages 1, 2 or 3), what your health is like, and if there are underlying or related conditions. A good treatment plan will also take into consideration your own health goals and what you would like to achieve.

There are two main treatment paths for high blood pressure: medication and lifestyle changes. Throughout this section of the book, we'll be diving into these in far more detail, but for now we'll give you a bit of an introduction into what these treatments can look like.

Medicines for high blood pressure

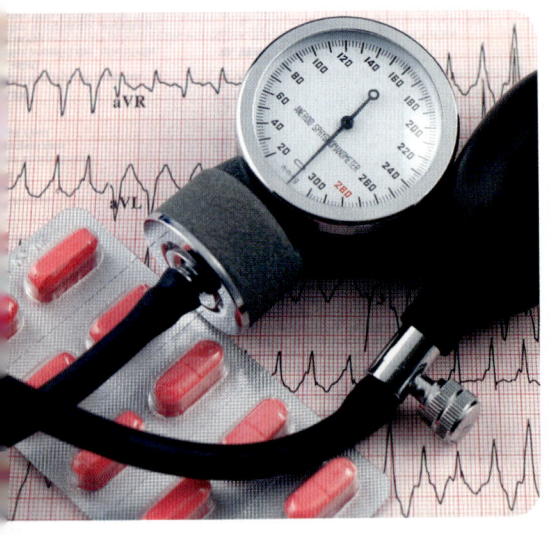

You may not be offered medication straight away for high blood pressure or it might be the first line of treatment – it all depends on your overall health, how advanced your hypertension is, and whether you have any signs of damage to any of your organs. Usually, medicine is offered as a treatment if you already have noticeable damage to the blood vessels in your heart, brain, kidneys or eyes; if you have heart disease or are at high risk of it developing; if you have kidney disease; or if you have diabetes. Medication can also be given if you have consistently very high blood pressure without any underlying or co-existing issues, especially if you are thought to be at high risk of going on to develop further health problems.

There are many different medications available to treat blood pressure in various ways, which we'll go through in more detail later on. However, you may not take just one type of blood pressure medication; there is some research that shows a

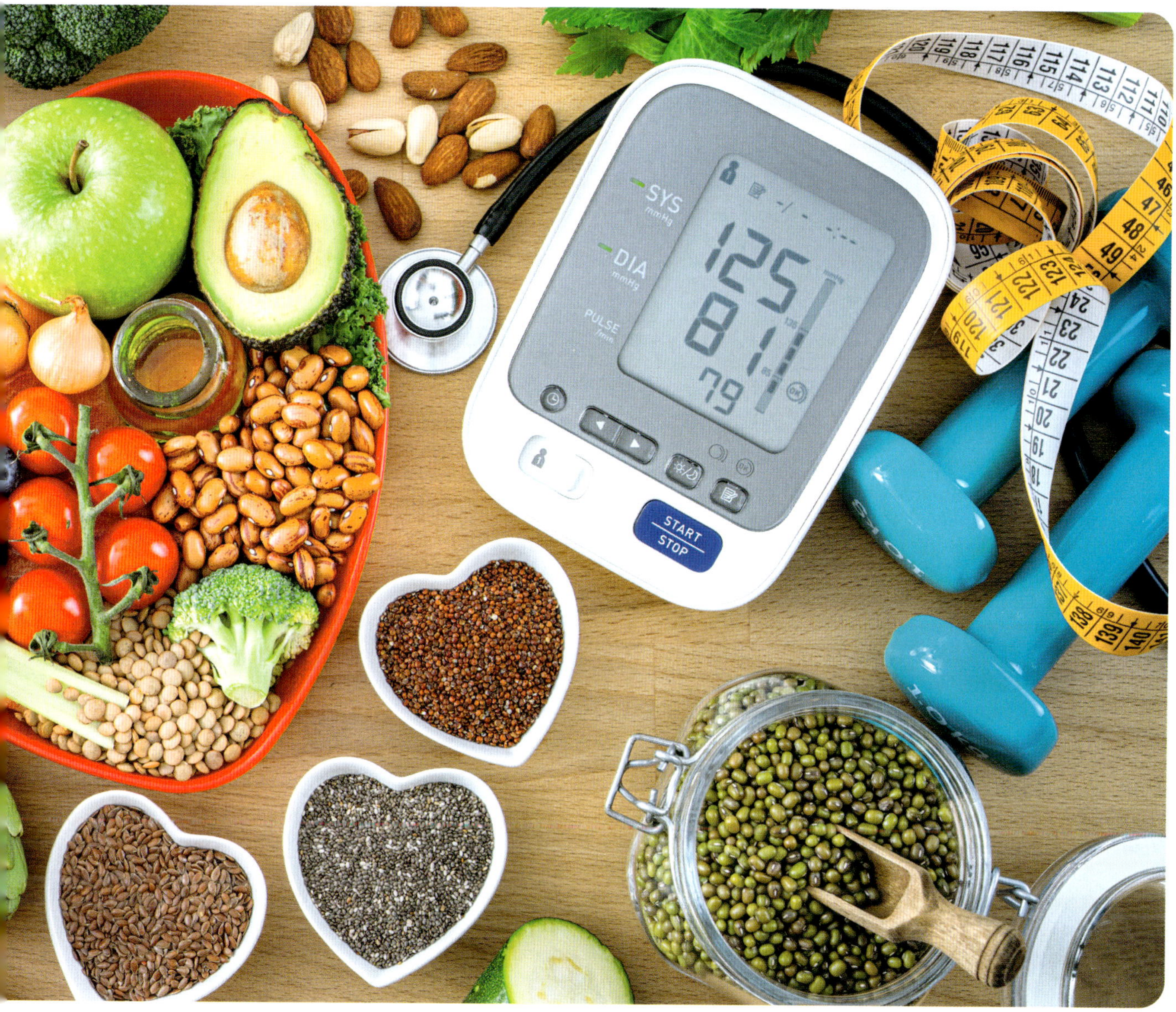

YOUR TREATMENT OPTIONS

combination of medications might be more effective. Some types of medication can't be taken by some people, whereas others can. And some are more effective than others for different people.

As a result, there is a certain amount of trial and error in finding the ideal medication. You'll be started with a standard dose of whatever treatment you are offered and then be asked to either take home blood pressure readings and submit them, or be seen regularly in person to have your blood pressure checked again. This is to determine if the medication is working. The dosage can then be tweaked to get better results. Once you are on the right dose of blood pressure medication, you will need to keep taking it as advised for a long time. If you stop it, your blood pressure could rise again, especially if the underlying causes or lifestyle risk factors have not been addressed. Sometimes, if your blood pressure stays under control for many years and you're making other lifestyle changes, it may be possible to reduce your dose or even come off the medication altogether. However, this is something that you will need to discuss with your doctor and not try to do yourself.

There are, inevitably, possible side effects of any medication you take, but the vast majority of people will be fine or have only mild side effects, and these are easier to manage than the potential health outcomes of uncontrolled high blood pressure.

If you have hypertension with no symptoms, as many people do, then it can be hard to come to terms with the fact that you need medication. This is a conversation to have with your doctor as they can advise you on whether lifestyle interventions will be enough, or whether you are going to need medication as well in order to get your blood pressure under control and reduce your risk of serious complications.

Lifestyle changes

There is a surprising amount you can do to get your blood pressure under control, and when you're

MANAGING HYPERTENSION

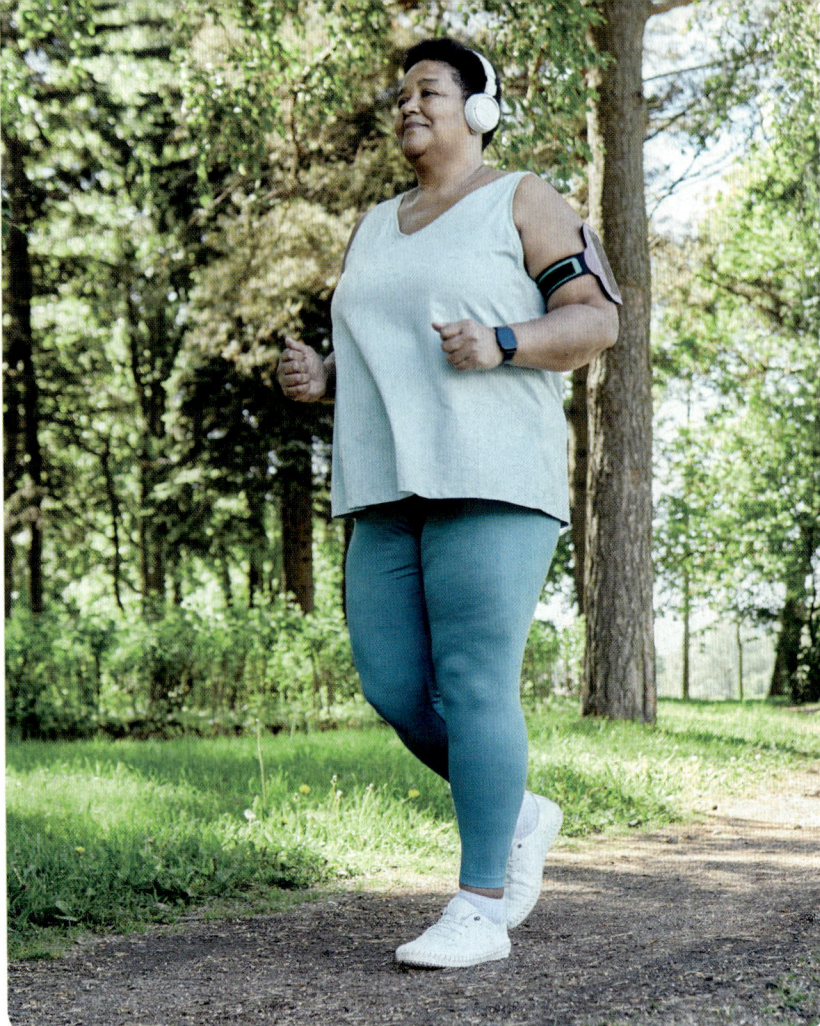

diagnosed, you will be given information about the options. It can be hard to commit to, what can be for some people, very big lifestyle changes. However, even small changes can be incredibly effective and start to bring your blood pressure down. Your doctor can refer you to different services to help you get started if you need them, or can work with you to come up with some lifestyle health goals to aim for.

If you are currently overweight or obese, then this will probably be the first area that will need to be addressed. It is not easy to lose weight and it's not something that will happen overnight, so it's important to break this down into smaller goals. In one study,[1] it was shown that blood pressure falls by around 2.5/1.5 mmHG for every kilogram (2.2 pounds) lost, so even committing to a small amount of weight loss can have a significant effect on your blood pressure. Being a healthy weight also helps control other health conditions, as well as reduce your risk for future complications.

Diet and exercise can help with weight loss, as well as with lowering your blood pressure. When it comes to food, the focus is on reducing your salt intake, which can mean getting used to reading labels on foods and not using table salt. You should instead focus on getting at least five portions of fruit and vegetables every day and reducing your intake of fatty foods. Eating in a healthy, balanced way can also help to lower your cholesterol, which is sometimes an issue alongside hypertension, as well as control other health conditions, like diabetes. Research shows that increasing your fruit and vegetable intake lowers blood pressure. When you're just getting started, it can be as important to focus on what you're adding into your diet as much as what you're trying to limit.

The other part of the puzzle is making sure that you get regular exercise. This can help with losing weight, if you need to, in addition to optimising heart function. If you don't currently exercise at all, the thought of this can be quite daunting, but you can build up slowly, with an aim to do some form of exercise five days a week for 30 minutes. This can be anything – you don't have to start running or join group classes, unless you want to. Gardening or vigorous house cleaning can get the heart rate up, as can brisk walking or swimming. The point is to start doing more than you're currently doing.

If you're a smoker, you'll be advised to quit and given some advice or signposted to support groups to help you with this. And if you drink alcohol, you should stay within the guidelines of no more than 14 units per week with several alcohol-free days each week. If your blood pressure is particularly high, you may be given a different limit for alcohol to help get it under control.

If your blood pressure is in the early stages of hypertension, then you may be given the opportunity to lower your blood pressure yourself through these lifestyle interventions. The hope is that making the right changes will be enough to bring it under control, without the need for medication. However, if you do need medication, a combined approach is often the most effective. Work with your medical team to come up with a plan that works for you and that you know you can commit to.

> "BEING A HEALTHY WEIGHT ALSO HELPS CONTROL OTHER HEALTH CONDITIONS"

[1] Influence of Weight Reduction on Blood Pressure: A Meta-Analysis of Randomized Controlled Trials, Hypertension, September 2003. [2] hopkinsmedicine.org.

YOUR TREATMENT OPTIONS

RESISTANT HYPERTENSION
What if you can't get your blood pressure under control?

There are some cases where a person's hypertension remains uncontrolled, despite intervention. This is called 'resistant hypertension'. There are various indications that you might have resistant hypertension, such as if you are taking three different medications at their highest dosages and yet your blood pressure remains above your goal. This might be because you actually have secondary hypertension that hasn't been picked up, meaning that there is an underlying cause for your hypertension, such as sleep apnoea, kidney failure or thyroid issues.

However, in around 75% of people with resistant hypertension,[2] there is no underlying reason for the resistance. It could be that the right combination of medication or dosage of medications hasn't been found yet, or that a person isn't always remembering to take them at the right time regularly enough. Or it could be that there are significant lifestyle contributors that haven't been addressed, or even that a person might be taking herbal supplements or other medicines that are impacting the effectiveness of the blood pressure treatment. It's not always straightforward.

SETTING HEALTH GOALS
Having clear targets to aim for can help you to stay motivated

When you first get diagnosed with high blood pressure and given a list of things you need to do, it can seem very overwhelming. Rather than trying to do everything at once, focus on one area at a time, starting with the thing that you feel needs the most work. Then set yourself some goals that will help you to stay focused on what you want to achieve. For example, if you decide that you want to target your diet first, then you can create some workable goals around that. These could be, for example, to increase your fruit and vegetable intake to five a day, to switch one unhealthy meal for a healthier one, or to cook a new recipe once a week, and so on. Once you get the hang of that and it becomes habit, you can then add in some more goals or look at another area in which you need to make changes. You're less likely to give up if you make a few new small habits at a time, rather than trying to overhaul everything in one go.

YOU'RE NOT ALONE
There are lots of support groups and services for people who have been diagnosed with hypertension.

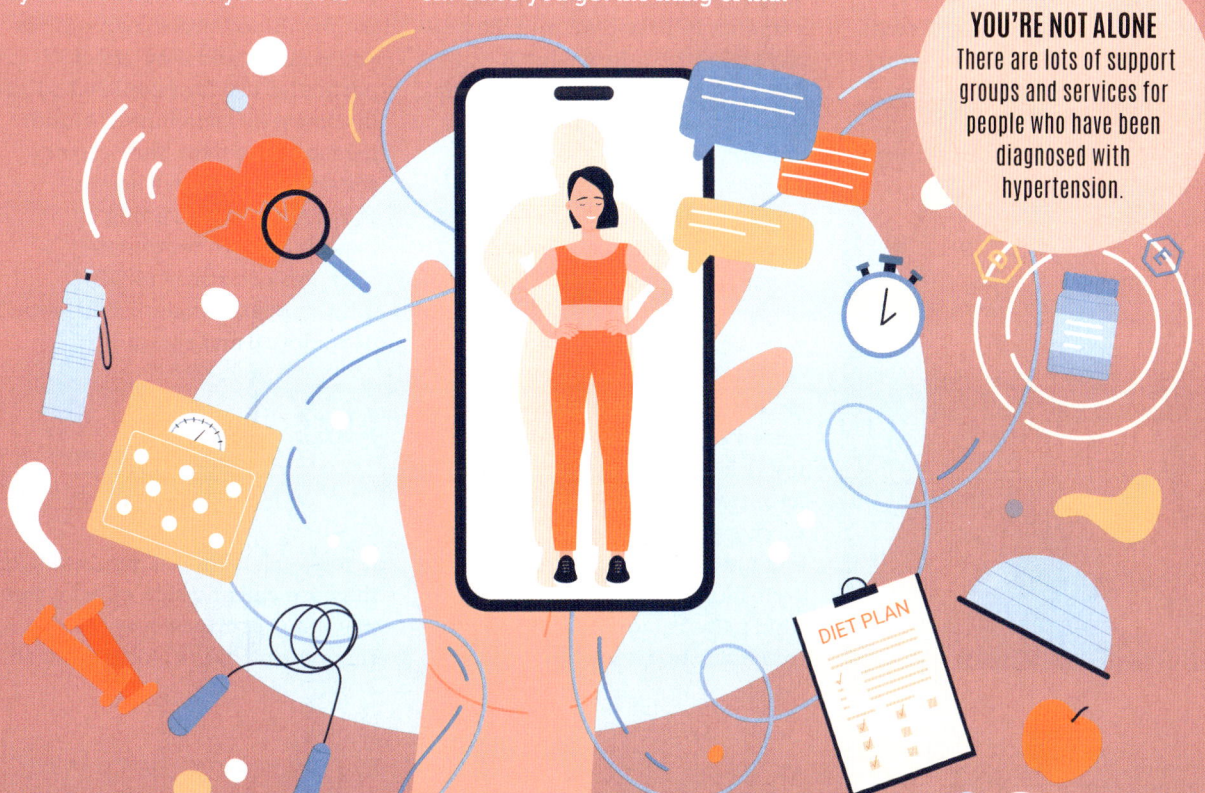

MANAGING HYPERTENSION

MEDICATIONS FOR HYPERTENSION

You may be advised to take a blood pressure medicine to help bring hypertension under control. We give you a rundown of the most common types

If you've been diagnosed with hypertension and advised to take medication, then you will be given one of the many different types of known blood pressure medicines that have been shown to be very effective. You may be advised to take more than one type, as they work together to bring blood pressure down. It can take some time to get the dosage and combination right for you, but you will be closely monitored to ensure that the medicine is working as it should.

Here we look at the key types of medicine used to treat hypertension that you may come across, along with how they work.

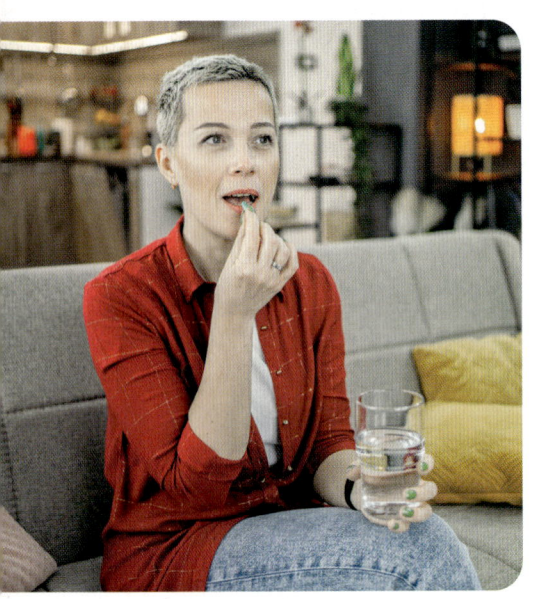

ACE inhibitors

ACE stands for angiotensin-converting enzyme, and ACE inhibitors are one of the most commonly prescribed types of blood pressure medicine. Angiotensin is a hormone in the body that causes blood vessels to narrow, raising blood pressure. It also plays a role in the way that the body retains sodium and fluid. There are different types of angiotensin in the body, which are named I, II, III and IV, and they all have slightly different jobs. Angiotensin II is the most relevant to hypertension, as it is the one that constricts blood vessels to increase blood pressure, increases the feeling of thirst and a desire for salt, stimulates the production of hormones that help the body retain salt, and alters the way the kidneys filter blood. While it's essential for our body, too much of it can contribute to raised blood pressure – some of the risk factors associated with hypertension cause angiotensin to increase. ACE inhibitors lower the amount of angiotensin, relaxing your blood vessels and allowing fluid to be removed more easily from your body, lowering blood pressure. An ACE inhibitor is often the first blood pressure medicine you will try, and they are of particular use for people who have diabetes, heart failure or kidney disease. However, they are not suitable for people who are pregnant, breastfeeding or planning to get pregnant.

Names of common ACE inhibitors are: enalapril, lisinopril, perindopril and ramipril.

NOT EVERYONE TAKES THEIR MEDICINE
It's estimated that 50-80% of hypertension patients do not take all their prescribed medicines.[1]

ARBs

If you can't take ACE inhibitors, or they are causing side effects, you may be prescribed angiotensin receptor blockers (ARBs) instead.

MEDICATIONS FOR HYPERTENSION

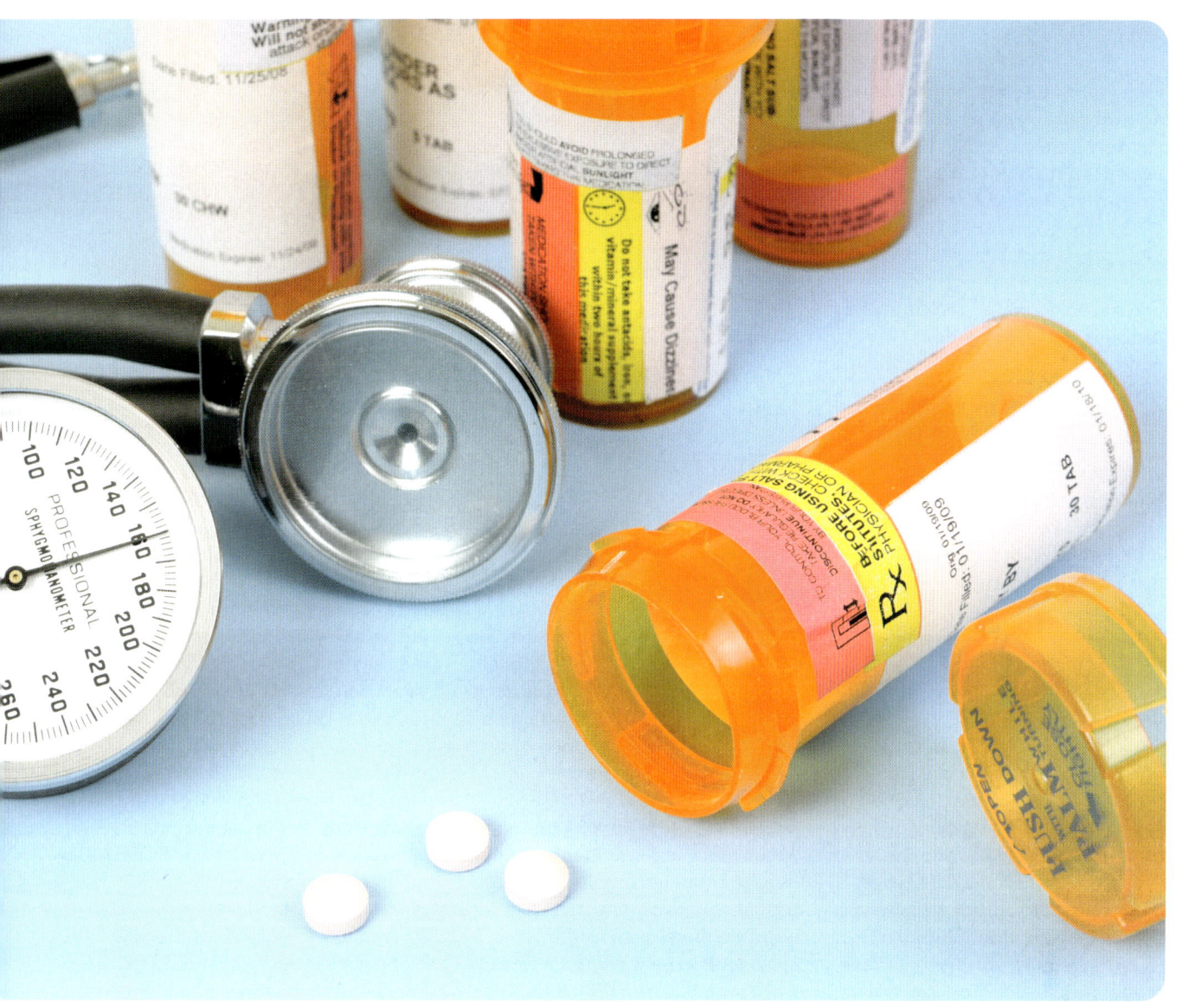

These work in a similar way, by blocking angiotensin II hormones in the body. Again, this helps the blood vessels to widen so that more blood can flow through, and more fluid can be released, lowering the pressure. They are often prescribed to people who have hypertension and are under 55 and not of African or Caribbean heritage. They are not suitable for people who are pregnant, breastfeeding or planning to get pregnant. They may also not be suitable if you have underlying health conditions or are already taking other medications, but your doctor will take all of this into consideration. While blood pressure medicines can be combined to give better effects, you would only take an ACE inhibitor or an ARB, as they work in similar ways. ARBs can, however, come as a combined pill with a calcium-channel blocker or diuretic included. ARBs are more effective in combination with a low-salt diet.

Names of common ARBs are: candesartan, irbesartan, losartan, valsartan and olmesartan.

CCBs

Calcium channel blockers (CCBs) work in a different way to either ACE inhibitors or ARBs. They do also help the blood vessels to relax and widen to give blood flow more space, however it is achieved through different means. CCBs are used to treat hypertension, as well as angina and abnormal heart rhythms. Calcium is an important mineral in the body, helping to build bones and teeth, regulating muscle contractions and helping blood to clot normally. One of calcium's roles is to help contract the heart muscles and the linings of blood vessels. Calcium passes into these cells through pores called ion channels. However, calcium buildup in the arteries can make the arteries become stiffer and less flexible, leading to hypertension. CCBs stop calcium from entering these channels and blocking the blood vessels.

There are two different types of CCB: dihydropyridines (usually

MANAGING HYPERTENSION

with names ending in 'pine') and non-dihydropyridines. The latter not only helps relax the blood vessels, but also helps control heart rhythms and heart rate. CCBs are an option for those who are pregnant or breastfeeding, as well as those with very high blood pressure and certain heart problems. They are often combined with ACE inhibitors or ARB. You will be told to avoid drinking grapefruit juice with certain CCBs, as this can react with the medicine and cause your blood pressure to suddenly drop.

Names of common CCBs are: amlodipine, diltiazem, felodipine, nifedipine and verapamil.

Thiazide diuretics

Diuretics, also called 'water pills', are a type of medicine that increase the production of urine, which helps your body to flush out excess salt and fluid. There are many health conditions where you could be prescribed diuretics, but in the case of hypertension, these would be thiazide diuretics, which help to reduce excess fluid from the blood, relieving the pressure on the blood vessels. Diuretics act directly on the kidneys, aiding them to take more salt and water out of the blood stream, to be released in urine. Diuretics also affect the blood vessel walls, helping them to relax and widen. They are usually prescribed if CCBs are not suitable or they're causing side effects. There are also other types of diuretics that can potentially be used if thiazide diuretics are not suitable. Diuretics may not be advisable for those with urinary, kidney or liver problems, diabetes or low potassium levels.

Common thiazide diuretics include: bendroflumethiazide, indapamide, chlortalidone, and cyclopenthiazide.

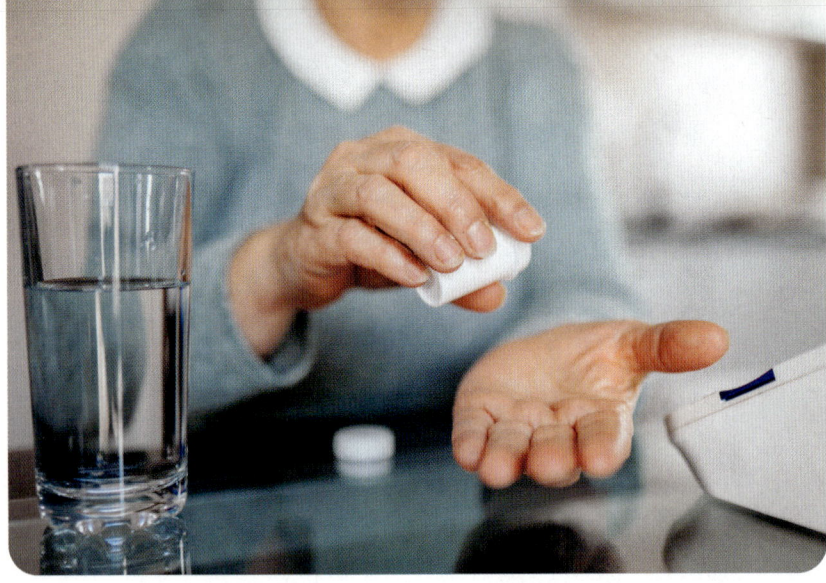

Non-standard medications

Sometimes you might need a little more help to lower your blood pressure, either due to underlying health issues, having very high blood pressure, having additional problems caused by hypertension, or because the normal medications are not suitable for you.

You might be offered medications like beta blockers, which are more commonly used to treat or recover from heart problems like angina, irregular heart rhythms, heart failure and heart attack. Beta blockers work by blocking adrenaline and noadrenaline, which make the heart beat faster and raise blood pressure. Beta blockers also block angiotensin II, making blood vessels widen and relax, which is why they are useful in reducing blood pressure. Alpha blockers also block the effects of adrenaline and noadrenaline, but are usually only used in cases where other treatments aren't working or are causing side effects. They are not normally part of a first line of treatment. Alpha blockers are also not often given to women, as they can cause stress incontinence.

You may also be offered a vasodilator, which dilates the blood vessels, making them wider to help blood flow through them more easily. They are also not usually a first line of treatment, as they can increase your heart rate and cause your body to hold on to excess fluid and water. Therefore, you would need other medications to control this.

Centrally acting hypertensive drugs, also known as central alpha antagonists, work directly on the brain. They target the part that controls blood pressure, reducing the force of your heartbeat and making your blood vessels relax. They can be used alongside other blood pressure medications and are usually only advised if other treatments are not bringing your blood pressure down enough.

As you can see, you have many options when it comes to blood pressure medication. Your doctor will explain what the right treatment option for you is. You will likely have to take the medication for several years to get your blood pressure under control and keep it there, if not longer, but most of them act quickly and you will have a lower risk of going on to develop more serious problems.

"SOMETIMES YOU MIGHT NEED A LITTLE MORE HELP TO LOWER YOUR BLOOD PRESSURE"

[1] Public Health England: Health Matters 2017.

MEDICATIONS FOR HYPERTENSION

SIDE EFFECTS

As with all medication, there can be some side effects to different blood pressure treatments

Most people cope well with blood pressure treatment. However, if you do experience side effects and they impact on your daily life, you may be able to change your dosage or try a different type of treatment. You should always tell your prescribing doctor of any side effects you notice. In the case of ACE inhibitors, the most common side effect is a persistent dry cough, but other possible side effects include dizziness, headaches, tiredness or a sudden drop in pressure when you stand up from a lying or seated position. Side effects of ARBs are similar, but they can also cause cold or flu-like symptoms (this isn't common, though). With both ACE inhibitors and ARBs, there is a very rare possibility of an allergic reaction, causing swelling around the mouth, face or throat.

If you're taking CCBs, or a combined pill with a CCB included, side effects can include a flushed face, swollen ankles, constipation, palpitations, ankle or foot pain, and skin rashes.

Thiazide diuretics can make you need to urinate more often, make you feel thirsty, cause an upset stomach or create a sensitivity to light. They can also cause muscle cramps, raised uric acid levels, raised blood sugar, erection problems in men, or dizziness.

CONTROLLED HYPERTENSION SAVES LIVES
A 10 mmHG reduction in systolic blood pressure reduces the risk of a major cardiovascular event by 20%.[1]

5 TIPS FOR BLOOD PRESSURE MEDICATION

If you've been prescribed blood pressure medication, taking it correctly helps its effectiveness

1. Take the right dosage
Double check that you understand how many pills you need to take and how many times a day. The medicine will only be effective if you follow your doctor's instructions.

2. Get into a good habit
It's best to take your medicines at the same time every day, so try to build it into your existing routine. This can help taking them become a habit, making you less likely to forget.

3. Be organised
Having a pill box can be handy for ensuring you've taken the right pills each day. You may also need to set timers at first until you get into the habit.

4. Read up
Do your research and understand what you're taking and how it works, as well as any side effects to watch out for. You should also check if there are any foods, drinks or herbal supplements that you need to avoid.

5. Stay positive
It can be hard to come to terms with taking a lot of medicine, especially when you feel well, but try to remember why you need them and the positive health outcomes you want to achieve.

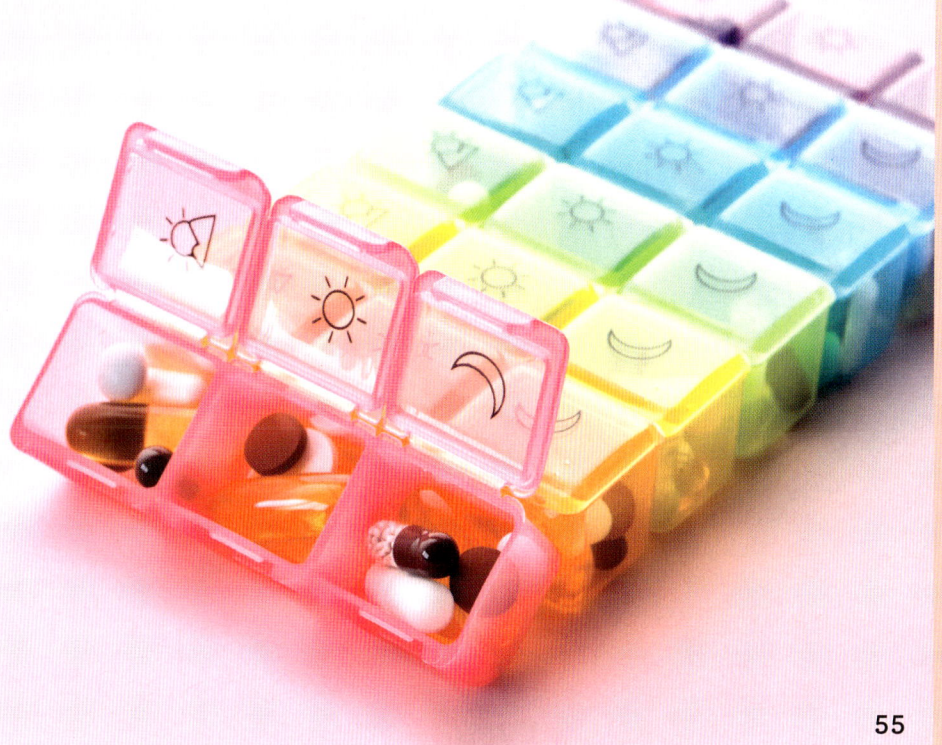

MANAGING
HYPERTENSION

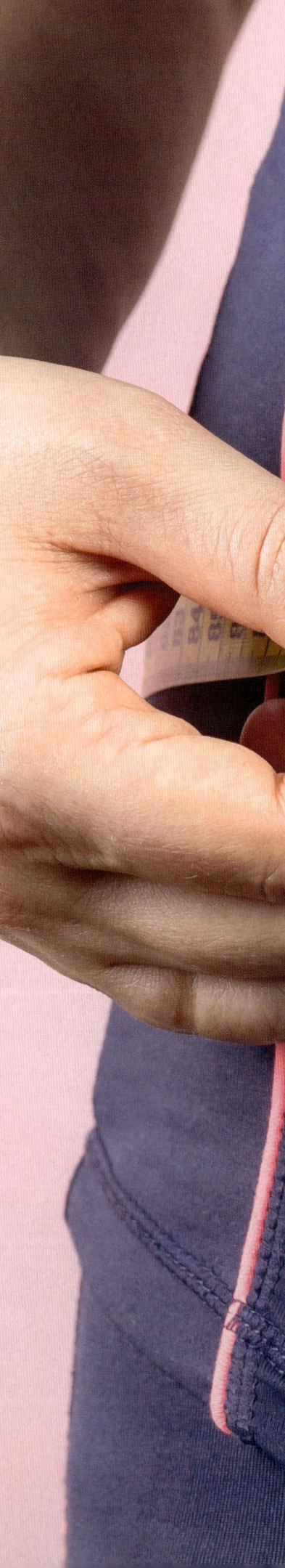

TAKE PHOTOS
Before and after photos can be a really great way to see how far you've come.

WEIGHT MANAGEMENT

Targeting or maintaining a healthy weight is one of the most important aspects of treating hypertension

If you are overweight or obese and are diagnosed with hypertension, then it's likely you will be advised to try and lose weight to get closer to a healthy weight range for your height. This is because we know that excess weight contributes to a higher blood pressure, and even losing a small amount of weight has a significant impact on reducing blood pressure. It's one of the most important lifestyle interventions, but it's not always easy.

There are lots of reasons why we might be overweight and some of these are easier to tackle than others. Sometimes our weight is impacted by other health issues that make it difficult to exercise, or cause us to hold on to more fat. We also live in a world where it can be easier to make less healthy decisions around food and exercise. In a regular supermarket, the amount of processed food on offer to tempt shoppers with taste and

WEIGHT MANAGEMENT

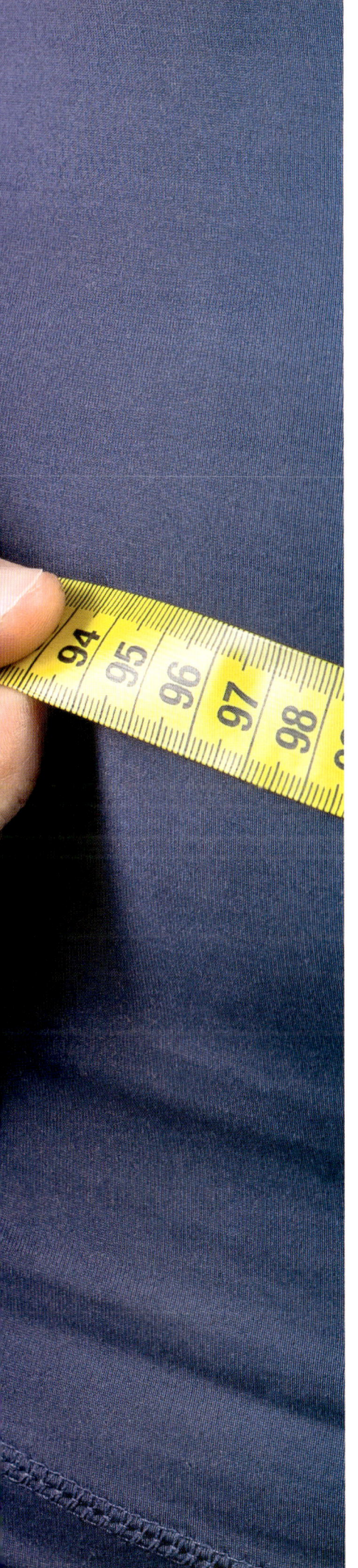

convenience can be hard to avoid. And when you're tired after a long day working, looking after family and everything else that modern life throws at us, the easy option – a ready meal, fast food or a takeaway, for example – is just one less thing to have to stress over. Some processed foods are also a lot cheaper and easier to access. Not to mention that they are engineered to make us want to eat them and overconsume them.

This isn't down to a lack of willpower; the modern food environment is not set up in a way that encourages healthy, balanced eating as the default. The same is true when it comes to exercise. Modern homes are very comfortable and filled with things we enjoy doing. We have on-demand streaming services with a plethora of television shows and movies at our fingertips; as well as video games and mobile games that are incredibly immersive and designed to draw us in and keep us playing. We might also drive more from place to place, sit down more at work, and work longer hours than ever before.

With all this happening around us, it's no wonder that it's easy to put on more weight than is ideal. However, when it's starting to impact your health, you need to make the conscious decision to do something to help yourself. It can be very overwhelming at first, especially if it means a big lifestyle change, but it could just save your life.

WEIGHT MANAGEMENT FOR HYPERTENSION

When you carry more weight – by which we mean mainly excess fat, as it's good to have plenty of lean muscle – than your body needs, the heart has to work much harder to pump blood around your body. If you also consume more fat, sugar and salt than is recommended, this can make the blood vessels stiffer, less flexible and narrower. This all increases your blood pressure, and it can be hard to get this under control. Medication can help to start to bring the pressure down, but it will be far more effective when combined with a lifestyle approach to weight loss. Tackling the underlying causes of high blood pressure means you can work towards being able to reduce, or maybe even stop, your medication in future years.

For people with an especially high BMI (over 30, unless you have a Black, Asian or ethnic minority background, in which case the threshold is lower), you may be able to access specific weight-loss programmes through local health services. Sometimes these programmes are also available to those whose BMI is lower, but have very high blood pressure or have diabetes. It's worth speaking to your regular doctor to ask about any referrals they can offer. This can be an online course, an in-person clinic or a partnership with a local gym, for example.

Even if you don't qualify for a referral, your doctor is a good starting point to find out what support and advice is available to you. Otherwise, there is plenty of weight-loss advice available online specifically for those who have hypertension if you need to find out more.

MANAGING
HYPERTENSION

GETTING STARTED

The first step to losing weight is usually the hardest. Most people who are overweight or obese are aware of this and probably know it's something they need to tackle, but don't know where or how to start. Don't be hard on yourself; this is a really common situation. It's a good idea to try to let go of everything you might have tried previously and give yourself a fresh start. So many of us have been on and off diets, especially those that offer quick fixes, only to find ourselves back where we started, or even in a worse place than where we started. The vast majority of named diets are overly restrictive, either in terms of calories or specific food groups, which is why they are hard to stick to. It's much better to move towards a sustainable, lifelong, healthy and balanced approach to food, complemented by regular physical exercise.

There is a specific diet plan that is tailored for people with hypertension called DASH – Dietary Approaches to Stop Hypertension. This is a way of eating that is designed to help reduce blood pressure and look after the heart. It's not specifically a weight-loss diet, as it focuses more on good nutrition, but many people will find that they do lose weight when following the principles of the diet. You may need to also calorie count, or at least be aware of your food intake, alongside following the principles of the DASH diet. We will look at this diet in more detail elsewhere, but its basic premise revolves around reducing salt, sugar and fat, while upping your intake of fruits and vegetables, wholegrains, low-fat dairy, lean meat and fish, healthy fats, nuts, beans and seeds.

This is an ideal and you may already eat close to this plan, or you might need to make a lot of changes. It's something to work towards, but not necessarily introduce from day one. The same goes for physical activity – the ideal is 150 minutes of moderate activity a week, which can be broken down into five days of 30 minutes' activity. However, if you currently don't exercise, then you won't want to jump right into this or you could risk injury. It's about being realistic of where your starting point is and thinking about setting some goals for what you'd like to achieve.

Many people find it useful to set a weight-loss goal. If you have a lot of weight to lose, it's much better

WEIGHT-LOSS SUPPORT GROUPS
Some people benefit from group-based help when trying to lose weight

We're all completely different when it comes to how we approach weight loss. Some people are very self-motivated and will be able to work towards a goal independently. Others, however, need a little more help and support. There are plenty of community groups based around weight loss, and these can help those who need extra accountability and advice. There are in-person groups available in your local area. These are either run by your local authority, a partner service or a commercial operation. They are all very different, so you will need to find the style that works for you. Some will ask you to 'weigh in' regularly and give certificates or badges when hitting milestones. This isn't for everyone, so ask about the structure of a group before joining. Other groups run more like courses to teach you about nutrition and physical activity, which can be great for grasping the basics and getting some fresh ideas. If in-person isn't something you're interested in, then there are also online support groups, which have the advantage of being more anonymous. You may find it easier to be honest in these environments, while still feeling like you have the support of others who understand what you're going through.

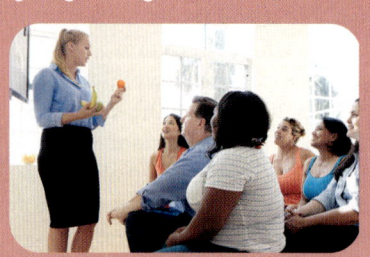

"THE GOAL IS TO CREATE SOMETHING FOR LIFE"

WEIGHT MANAGEMENT

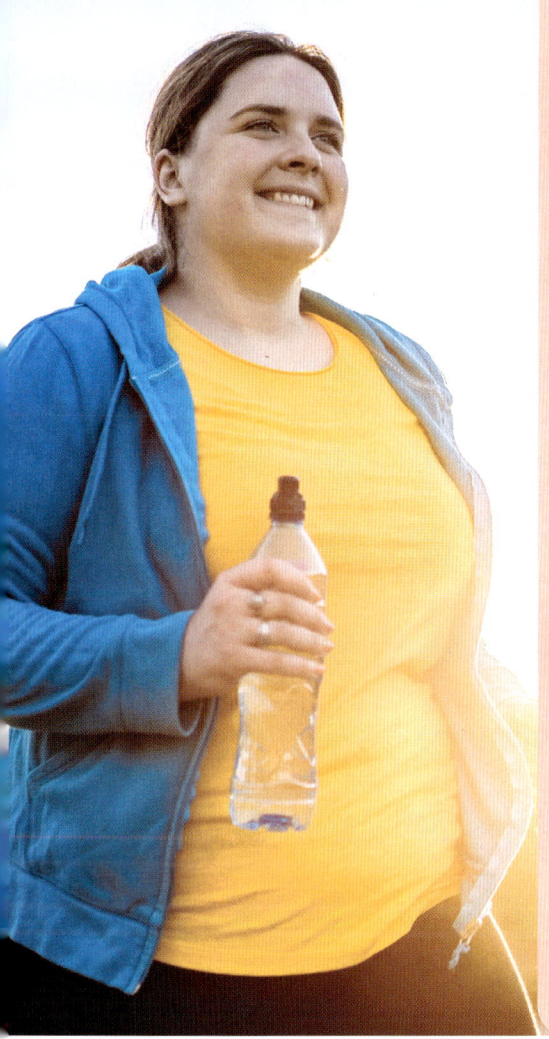

TRACKING FOOD AND EXERCISE

Keeping a log of your day-to-day lifestyle can help you stay focused on your goals

Analysis from the Office of National Statistics in 2018 revealed that a third of people in the UK underestimate how many calories they're eating – by as much as 1,000 calories. This discrepancy is fuelled by a lack of understanding around nutrition, snacking on the go, and nutritional information not being clearly labelled. When you're trying to lose weight, a useful task is to start tracking what you eat and how much exercise you do. It can be a good idea to track a couple of normal days before you start making any changes. This can help you identify the areas that you need to tackle first. It's up to you how you track. There are some great apps available that scan different foods, and count up calories and other nutritional metrics, as well as take into account your daily movement. You can also just use a pen and paper tracker, or make notes in a small notebook. You may prefer not to count calories, but even just writing down what you eat and when, without any values, can be helpful for seeing what volume of foods you're eating, whether you're getting enough fruit and vegetables, and if you're prone to snacking at certain times.

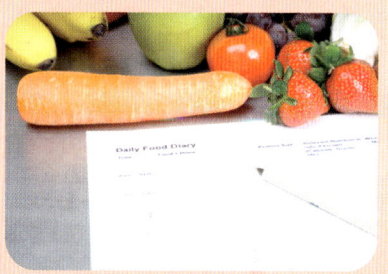

for your focus and motivation to set interim goals along the way towards your ultimate target. A sensible amount of weight to lose is around 0.5-1 kilogram (one or two pounds) a week. You may lose a lot more than this at first, depending on how many changes you make to your lifestyle, but this should taper off as you adjust to your food and exercise plan. Losing small increments of weight can help you to keep it off in the long term, as can educating yourself around nutrition and exercise. Thinking in terms of a 'diet' can suggest that it's a short-term fix before returning to normal, but the goal is to create something that is sustainable for life.

REWARD YOURSELF
Decide on incentives for when you reach a goal, as this will help you to stay motivated.

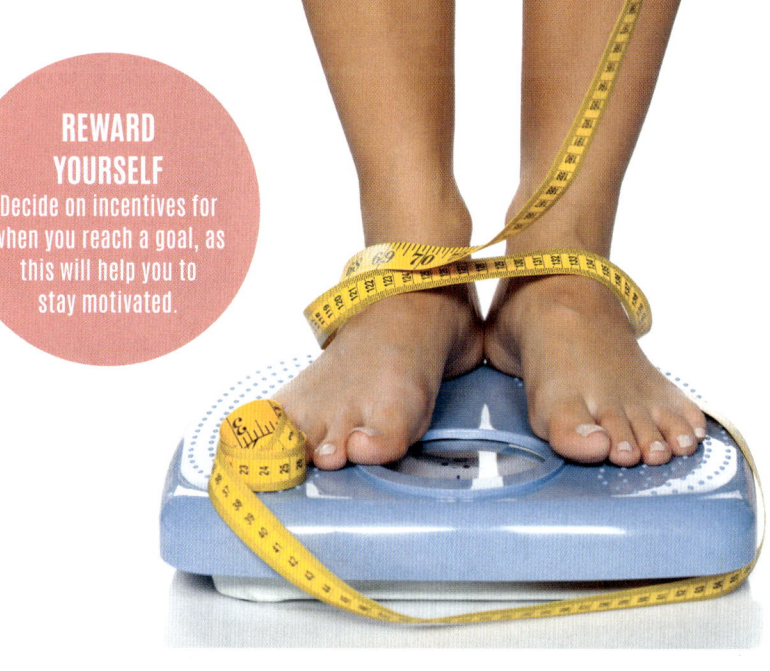

Images Getty

MANAGING
HYPERTENSION

SUSTAINABLE WEIGHT-LOSS TIPS

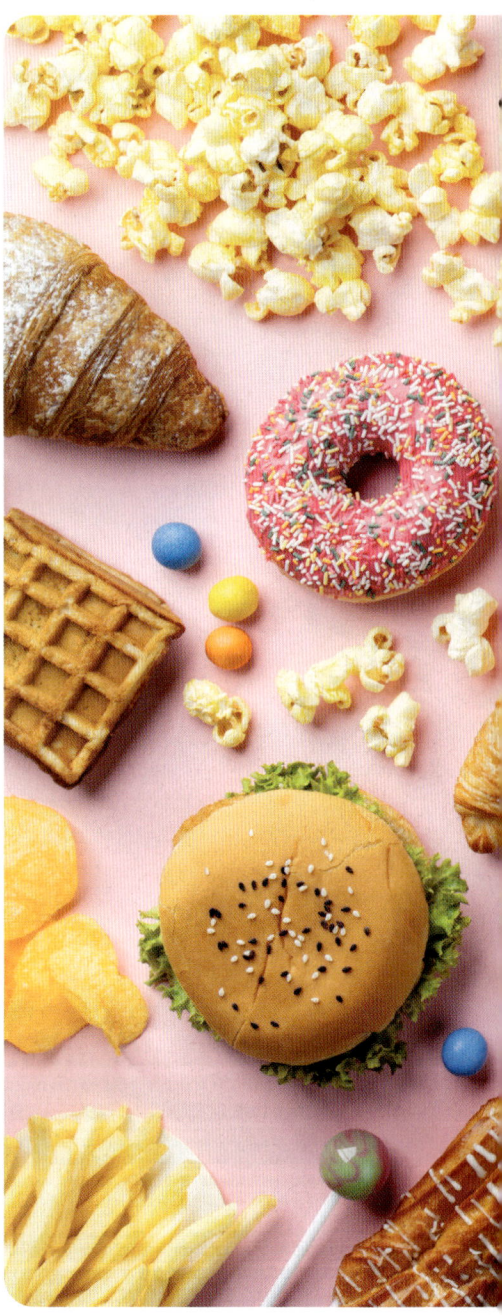

A good way to start losing weight is to learn more about the foods you eat most often. This might mean reading labels or looking at the construction of a typical meal for you. You could be shocked to learn the nutritional values of some of your favourite foods! Education is really important. Being on a 'diet' can so often feel like punishment, which makes it much harder to stick to. However, if you learn what certain foods do to your body, both positively and negatively, it empowers you to make better choices that help to fuel and nourish your body, instead of harming it.

Try to stick to introducing one big change at a time. You may prefer to focus, at first, on adding in lots of nutritious foods to your meals – an extra portion of fruit as a snack, a big side salad with lunch and a colourful selection of vegetables with dinner. You could also start to change how you cook your foods, so instead of frying, you could bake; instead of using butter, you could switch to a drizzle of quality olive oil. Try to slow down when eating as well, being mindful about each bite and learning to recognise when you've had enough. Reduce your portion size, so that you're still eating all the same foods, just slightly less of them.

When you've got to grips with these kinds of changes, you might feel ready to start looking at the quality of the foods you're eating

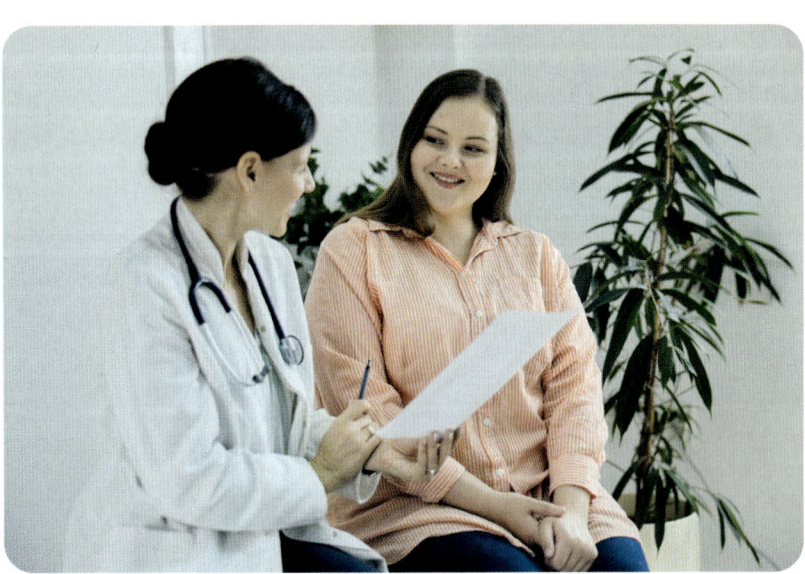

"BUILD HEALTHY HABITS INTO YOUR LIFE IN A WAY THAT FITS YOU AND YOUR FAMILY"

and begin to make healthier choices or reduce your intake of less-healthy options. Don't over-restrict, as you'll just end up craving what you 'can't' have and this can lead to overindulgence. Everything is okay in moderation. Maybe you decide to only have chocolate at the weekend, or you drink alcohol on fewer days a week. Sometimes it's best to start with some simple swaps, so that you can follow your usual pattern but with effective changes. Switch white bread to wholegrain, full-fat dairy to low fat, choose a leaner cut of meat, have porridge instead

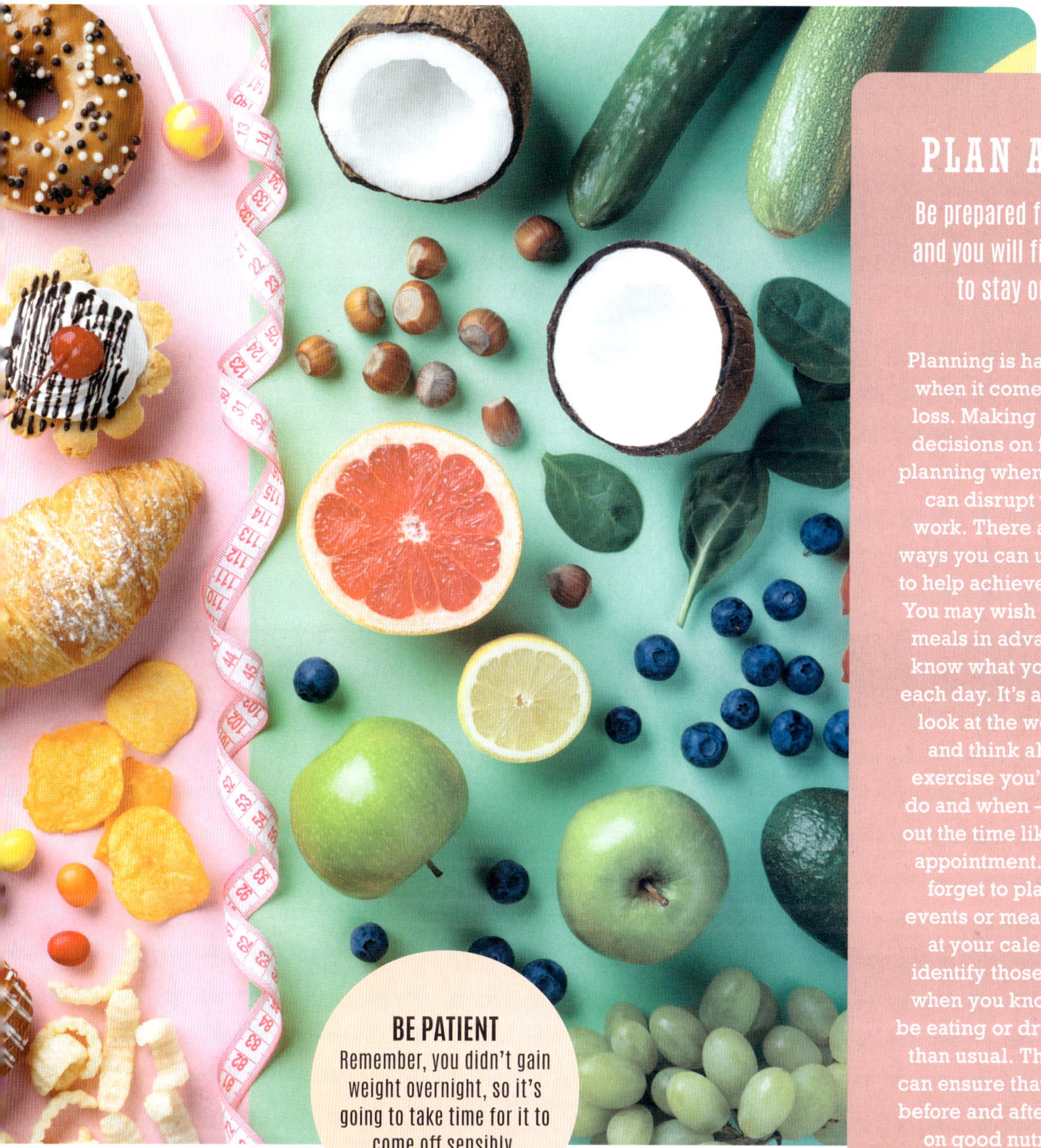

WEIGHT MANAGEMENT

BE PATIENT
Remember, you didn't gain weight overnight, so it's going to take time for it to come off sensibly.

of cereal, use herbs and spices instead of salt.

Whatever you decide to change, you should ensure that you are working around your lifestyle. There's little point planning elaborate meals if you don't have the time to cook them, or planning to go to the gym every day when you have a busy job. You are more likely to succeed if you can build healthy habits into your life in a way that fits you and your family. This might mean sticking to very simple meals in the week – jacket potato with healthy toppings, a chicken salad, grilled fish with potatoes and vegetables, soup – or you might use time at the weekend to do some batch cooking to help you in the week. When it comes to exercise, can you use the daily commute to get some activity in? Could you walk in your lunch break or spend a few hours gardening at the weekend?

Don't forget that you're not alone. Losing weight can be hard work, but every step you take towards your goal is helping to get your blood pressure under control and reducing your risk of serious health problems.

PLAN AHEAD
Be prepared for anything and you will find it easier to stay on track

Planning is half the battle when it comes to weight loss. Making last-minute decisions on food, or not planning when to exercise, can disrupt your hard work. There are various ways you can use planning to help achieve your goals. You may wish to plan your meals in advance so you know what you're eating each day. It's also useful to look at the week ahead and think about what exercise you're going to do and when – then block out the time like any other appointment. And don't forget to plan for any events or meals out. Look at your calendar and identify those occasions when you know you will be eating or drinking more than usual. This way you can ensure that in the days before and after, you focus on good nutrition and drinking plenty of water. One event won't hinder your progress if you're on track around it, and it's important that you enjoy your life. This is a long-term lifestyle and not a short-term fix.

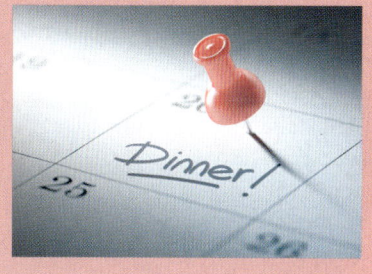

MANAGING
HYPERTENSION

STRESS AND HYPERTENSION

We might associate high stress with high blood pressure, but that's not always the case. However, managing stress can help to control other risk factors

Many of us think that stress, especially long-term stress, is a direct cause of high blood pressure. It makes sense, but actually research shows that there is no evidence that stress contributes to hypertension. That's not to say it doesn't have an impact on your blood pressure, but this tends to be a short-term thing, with blood pressure returning to normal once the stress has passed.

However, it's not uncommon for stress and hypertension to coexist. If you have stress for a long time, or if you already have hypertension, then even a short-term rise in blood pressure needs to be managed. Being under stress can also lead to an increase in lifestyle habits that we know are a risk factor for hypertension, meaning that stress can be more common among those with high blood pressure. One study, aiming to estimate the prevalence of stress in hypertensive patients, found that over 84% experienced some level of stress, yet less than 3% of these patients asked for any professional help.[1]

As such, it's important to learn to recognise the signs of stress and how to manage it alongside managing your hypertension. Luckily, many of the treatment options for hypertension can help to reduce stress, and many of the interventions for stress can help with controlling blood pressure.

What is stress?

Stress is a natural reaction to situations that make us feel under pressure or under threat. Everyone has a different threshold for what makes them feel stressed. Usually there is an element of feeling out of control or helpless, unable to change a situation in which we feel stress. For example, workplace stress is quite common, with people feeling under pressure to perform, meet deadlines and work as part of a team. Other causes of stress can be when unexpected things happen, such as a flat tyre or a missed bus. Parents and carers can feel a lot of stress when having to cope with the pressures of looking after others a lot of the time. Other common reasons why people might

COMMON PROBLEM
A 2023 survey of adults in 142 countries found that 37% of people are experiencing a lot of stress.[2]

"IT'S IMPORTANT TO LEARN SIGNS OF STRESS"

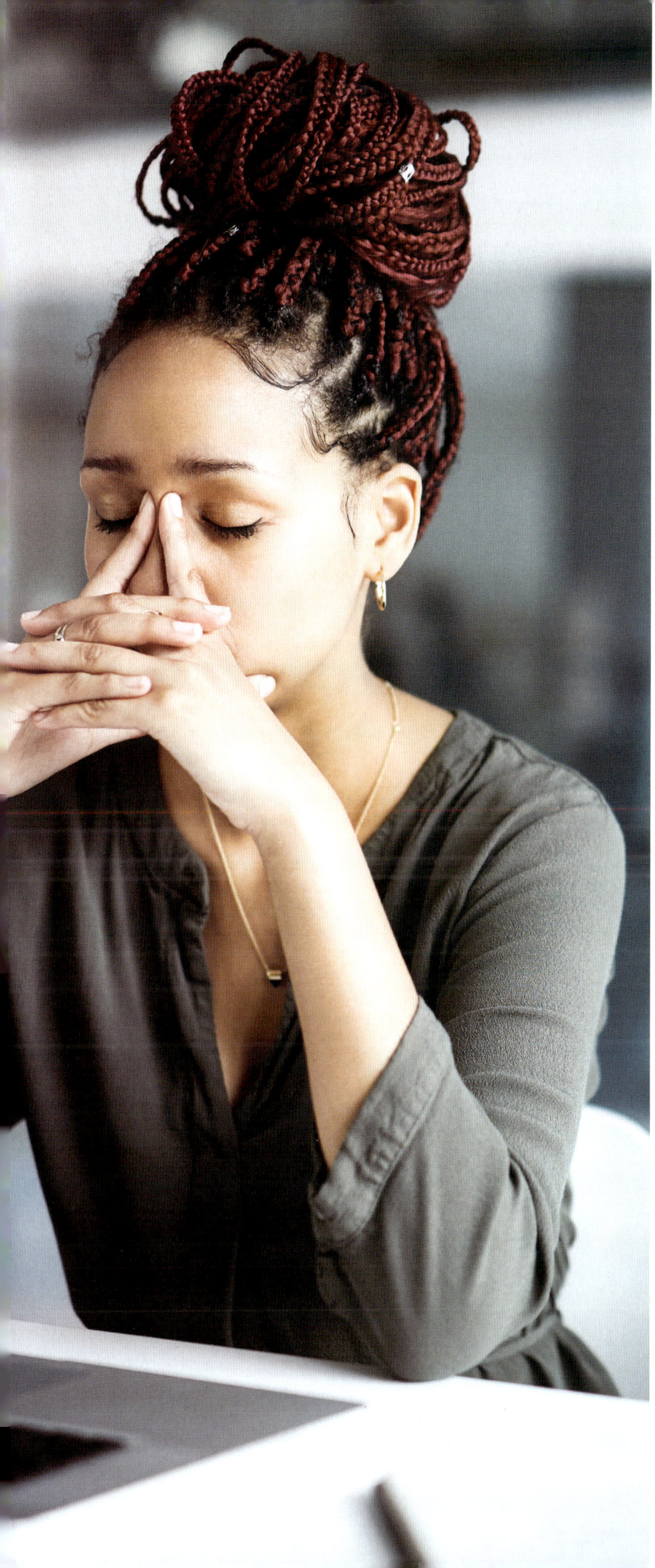

STRESS AND HYPERTENSION

feel stressed include having financial problems or suffering a bereavement. Some people also feel stressed with global issues, such as the climate crisis or natural disasters.

A little stress can be quite good for us. For example, if you're feeling stressed about meeting a deadline, the stress can help you to feel more motivated and focused to get the project done in time. However, too much stress, long-term stress, or very intense stress, is more of a problem. Intense periods of stress are called 'acute stress' and this is usually triggered by a specific event that is traumatic or difficult to process. This acute stress starts from the moment of the event and can last until you come to terms with the event. Long-term stress is 'chronic stress' and this is when you feel stressed a lot of the time for a longer period of time. It might go away and come back again, or be there constantly. This is more common in situations where there is an underlying reason for your stress related to your lifestyle, for example, if you're caring for someone or have worries about money.

Stress can then lead to the development of mental health problems such as anxiety and depression, and some mental health conditions can also cause stress. For example, if you have anxiety, you may find that you feel stressed about things more often than usual. Stress can cause both physical and mental symptoms (which you can read about in our box on page 65).

Stress and blood pressure

When we're under stress, our body perceives a threat and reacts accordingly. The brain triggers the release of adrenaline, which causes your heart rate to speed up

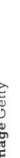

MANAGING HYPERTENSION

and your blood pressure to rise. This is a short-term reaction to help us cope with the stressful situation we're dealing with. And when that stress passes, both of these metrics should return to normal. Chronic stress can mean that our heart rate and blood pressure are being raised more often, with less chance to recover in between.

The biggest problem with stress, in relation to hypertension, is that it can cause an increase in the other risk factors that we know cause high blood pressure. For example, many people who are very stressed will turn to smoking or drinking more than usual to help them cope with the stress, both of which are direct causes of hypertension. You may also find that you eat more than normal, which can lead to weight gain – another cause of high blood pressure. Even if you're not eating more, you may opt for junk food or convenience food, which can mean you're consuming more salt, fat and sugar, again contributing to a rise in blood pressure.

It can be difficult to find the time and motivation to exercise when you are under a lot of stress. If you're working long hours, for example, which is making you feel stressed and under pressure, you're also not getting enough time outside or doing physical activity. Stress can also impact on your sleep, which can contribute to low energy and low motivation.

So, while there isn't yet a definitive cause-and-effect link between stress and hypertension (though there is research ongoing in this area), you can see how closely linked hypertension management and stress management are. If you have a lot of stress, then you should try to manage this as best you can.

Learning to manage stress

Stress management is mostly about lifestyle intervention. Getting outside in nature can help relieve stress, so see if you can work a daily walk into your schedule. This could be as part of a commute, a lunch-time walk, or a family outing at the weekend. As regular exercise is a great way to reduce stress, you can easily combine these two interventions to get the biggest benefit.

It's also important to prioritise when you're feeling stressed. You might feel overwhelmed and that you have a lot to do. Try to make a list of what's worrying you and categorise these worries into the things you absolutely have to do; the things you can delegate; and the things that can wait. This can help you gain a little more perspective and feel less stressed. Try to include some lifestyle interventions within your priorities, especially if you already have hypertension. This can be making sure you always eat healthy meals, even if they need to be quick and easy – keep things simple, and focus on getting enough fruits and vegetables. Make sure you give yourself time to switch off at night so that you can get enough sleep to help you cope with the stress as best you can. You may also want to try putting aside a few minutes a day to do some breathing exercises (we have supplied one for you in the box on page 65) or plan in some regular yoga or meditation.

The most important thing is to recognise when you're under stress and to put strategies in place to manage this. The aim is to ensure your coping mechanisms do not affect your hypertension, as this will leave you at risk of further health complications.

> "STRESS CAN CAUSE AN INCREASE IN THE OTHER RISK FACTORS THAT CAUSE HIGH BLOOD PRESSURE"

GET HELP
If you are finding stress unmanageable and you can't get it under control, seek help from a doctor.

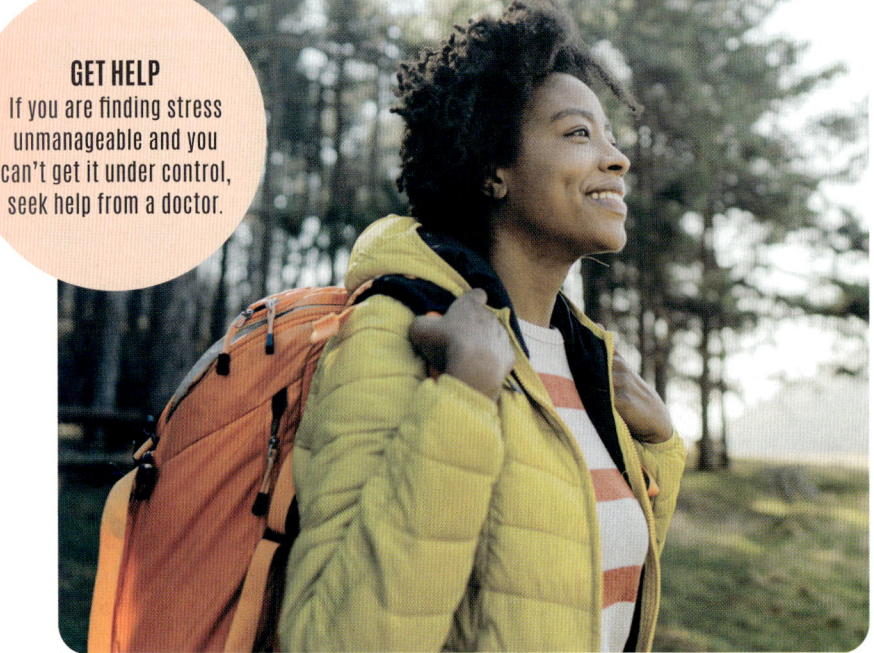

[1] A lay epidemiological study on coexistent stress in hypertension: Its prevalence, risk factors, and implications in patients' lives. Journal of Family Medicine and Primary Care, 2019. [2] Gallup Global Emotions Report 2024.

STRESS AND HYPERTENSION

SYMPTOMS OF STRESS

When you're under a lot of stress, you might feel both physical and mental symptoms

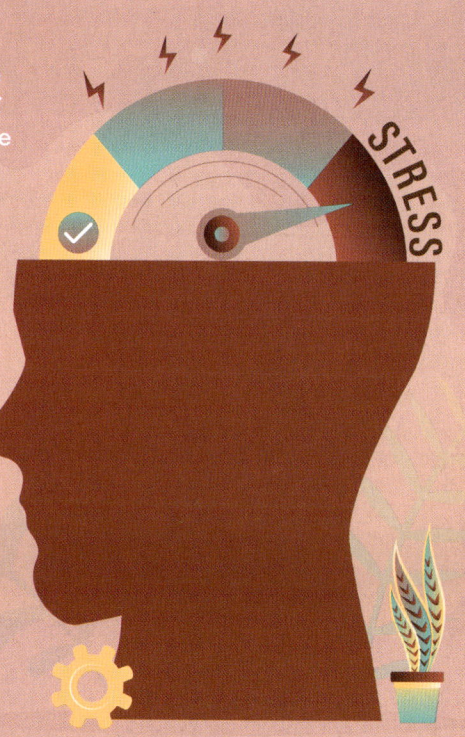

Everyone reacts to stress differently and you may have some, but probably not all, of these symptoms when you are feeling stressed.

Physical symptoms
- Pain in your chest
- Increase in heart rate
- Tight headaches across both sides of the head
- Dizziness
- Stomach problems
- Feeling tense or tight
- Aches and pains

Mental symptoms
- Being irritable or angry
- Feeling overwhelmed
- Feeling anxious of worried
- Finding it hard to make decisions
- Difficulty concentrating or staying focused
- More forgetful than usual
- Unable to switch off racing thoughts

Long-term exposure to stress can lead to other mental health problems, like anxiety or depression. If you already have an underlying mental health condition, then stress can make it worse.

CALMING BREATH EXERCISE

If you're feeling stressed, try this breathing exercise to help you feel calmer

When you're feeling overwhelmed and stressed, the best thing you can do is extract yourself from the current situation and take a few moments to calm yourself down. It helps if you can go to a place where you won't be disturbed and it is quiet, where you can sit and relax. If you're not able to do this in the moment, or if you're feeling a level of stress all the time, then you could try this at bedtime before you go to sleep instead.

There are lots of breathing patterns that can help you feel calmer. They all work in the same way: they make you intentionally notice your breath and focus on it, which can still your thoughts and help you to be more present.

One technique that you can try is called 4-7-8 breathing. When you are somewhere calm and quiet, try this:

- **Inhale deeply through your nose for 4 seconds**
- **Hold your breath for 7 seconds**
- **Exhale slowly through your mouth for 8 seconds**
- **Repeat**

This method can help to reduce feelings of anxiety, improve sleep, and also lower your heart rate and blood pressure.

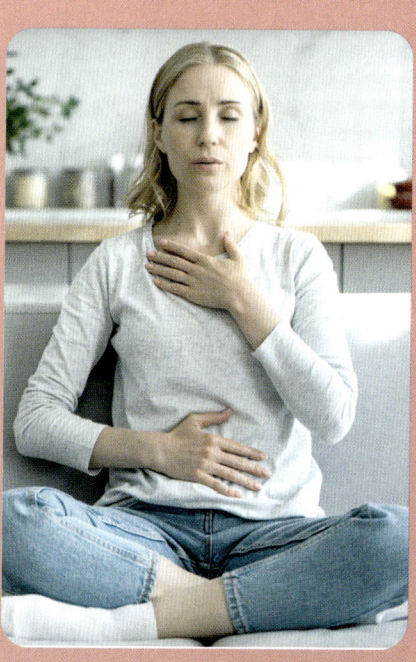

MANAGING
HYPERTENSION

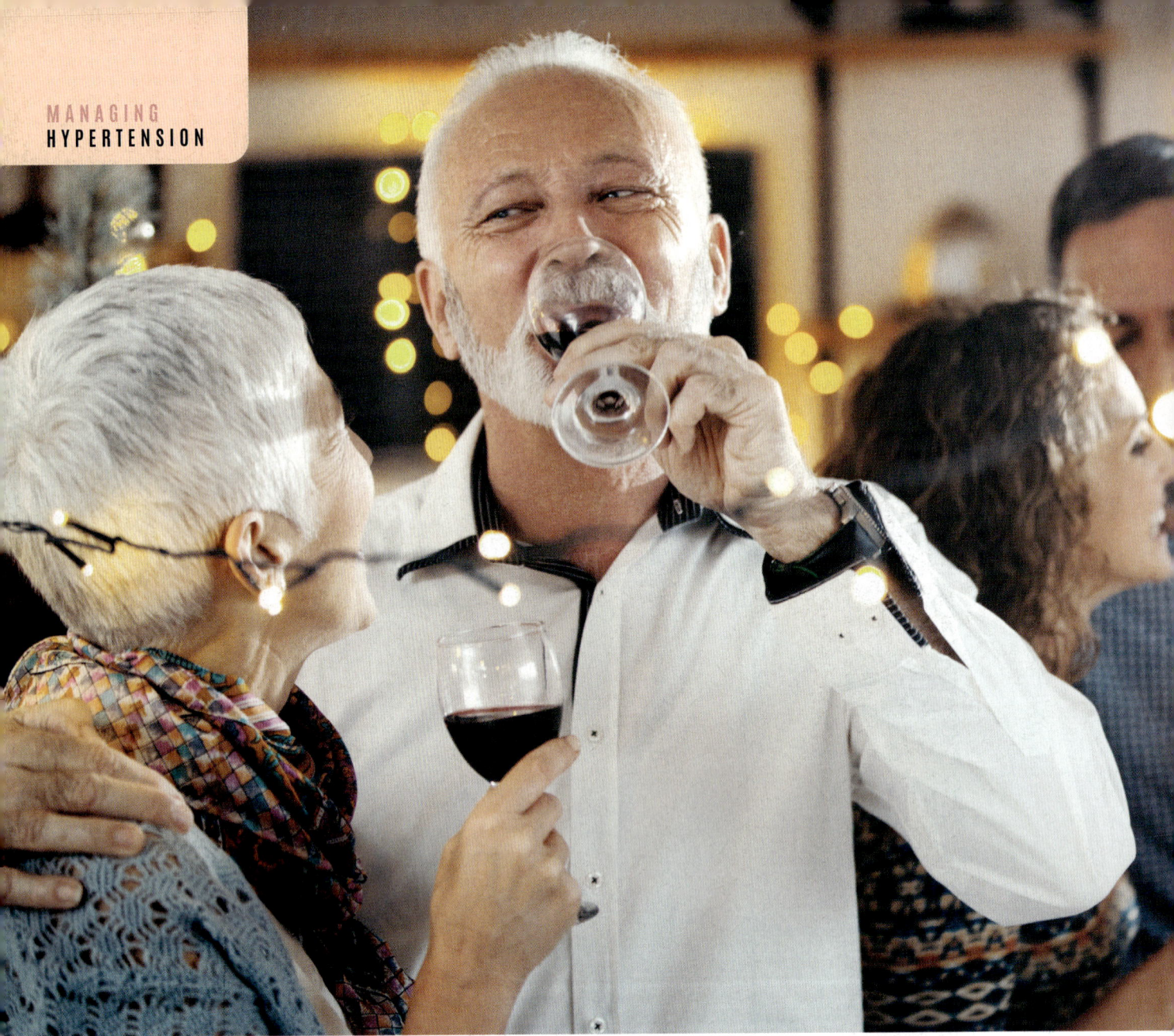

MANAGING ALCOHOL CONSUMPTION

If you have high blood pressure, you may need to cut down on – or even cut out – alcohol as part of your treatment plan

Some causes of hypertension are unmodifiable, meaning that they are risk factors that we can't do anything about. However, some causes are behavioural, which means they are within our control to change.

Drinking alcohol is a preventable cause of high blood pressure. There is very good evidence that drinking alcohol significantly heightens the risk of developing hypertension, heart problems and having a stroke.

A report released in 2023[1] analysed seven studies covering more than 19,000 adults in the USA, Korea and Japan, and found that there was a definite link between increases in systolic blood pressure and the number of

MANAGING ALCOHOL CONSUMPTION

THE LINK BETWEEN ALCOHOL AND HIGH BLOOD PRESSURE

So we know that drinking too much alcohol raises your blood pressure – in fact, it's one of the most common health problems related to alcohol. While even one drink can lead to a short-term rise in blood pressure, regularly drinking too much alcohol leads to hypertension, where your blood pressure rises and stays high. If you drink heavily, this can lead to severe hypertension.

When you drink alcohol, especially if it's more than the recommended amount on a regular basis, it puts a lot of pressure on your blood vessels and causes them to become narrower. If you have one drink a day, this is enough to increase the risk of developing high blood pressure. And if you have already been diagnosed with hypertension, you will increase your risk of it becoming more severe. This leads to an increased risk of heart disease, stroke and an irregular heartbeat. For those who already have an irregular heartbeat (called arrhythmia), alcohol can make the condition worse. Overconsumption of alcohol can also lead to alcoholic cardiomyopathy, which can lead to heart failure.

It's not just the direct effect of the alcohol that impacts on your blood pressure, but the side effects of it too. Alcohol is quite high in calories, so if you drink a lot, it can lead to weight gain. We know that being overweight is highly associated with hypertension. Some drinks are more calorific than others. A pint of beer, for example, could be around 200 calories, and a standard (175ml) glass of wine could be around 150 calories. You can see how easily this can build up if you have a few. Plus, these liquid calories don't replace food, so you're likely to want to eat more than usual or make less heathy choices. You might then feel groggy and tired the next day, meaning that you're less likely to make good food decisions or want to get out and exercise.

MEASURE IT OUT
It's easy to overfill drinks at home, so make sure you accurately measure when pouring.

alcoholic drinks consumed per day. It also showed that even those who drank one drink a day had higher blood pressure compared to those who didn't drink at all, and that there was a continuous increase in blood pressure over time when alcohol was regularly consumed. None of the study participants had hypertension at the start, but those who had higher starting numbers were impacted more by alcohol intake than those who started with lower numbers.

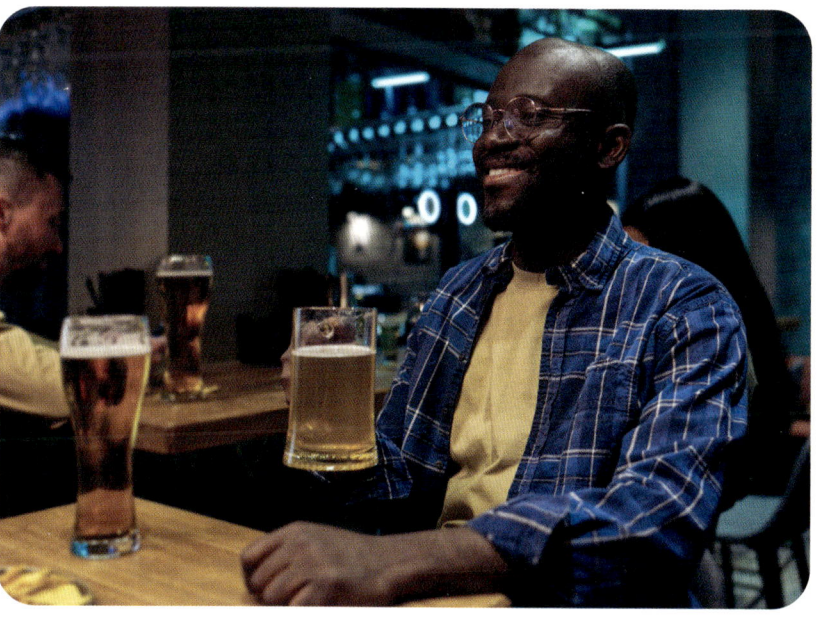

67

MANAGING HYPERTENSION

HOW MUCH ALCOHOL?

We live in a world where it can be hard to stop drinking, especially if your social life revolves around having alcohol or you find it relaxing. The most common question for most people is, 'How much is safe for me to drink?'. Sadly, the answer is that there is no recommended 'safe' limit. The best amount of alcohol for the human body is zero.

However, that's not practical advice for those who enjoy and wish to continue to enjoy a drink. Therefore, there are guidelines that are based around how much is considered 'low risk' rather than 'safe'. For all adults, men and women, the guidelines in the UK state that those who regularly drink more than 14 units a week are at higher risk of health problems. And this should be spread out over at least three days or more, with alcohol-free days every week. Guidelines vary in other countries, but most set a suggested limit. In the USA, drinking in moderation is considered to be a limit of two drinks or less a day for men and one drink or less a day for women.

It can be hard to visualise what 14 units looks like in a week. It's roughly equivalent to six standard glasses of wine or pints of beer, depending on the strength of the drink. Drinking more than six units in six hours is what is classed as 'binge drinking' – which is less than three standard glasses of wine or three pints in one sitting. This can come as a surprise to many people who might not consider themselves as drinking too much. Many of us will drink more than the 14 units in a week and even binge drink every so often, without thinking of it as a problem.

When you are diagnosed with high blood pressure, you will be asked about your alcohol consumption. If it's above the amount stated in the guidelines, then you'll be advised to cut down. If you have severe hypertension or are high risk for related health conditions, you may be advised to stop altogether.

> "WE LIVE IN A WORLD WHERE IT CAN BE HARD TO STOP DRINKING"

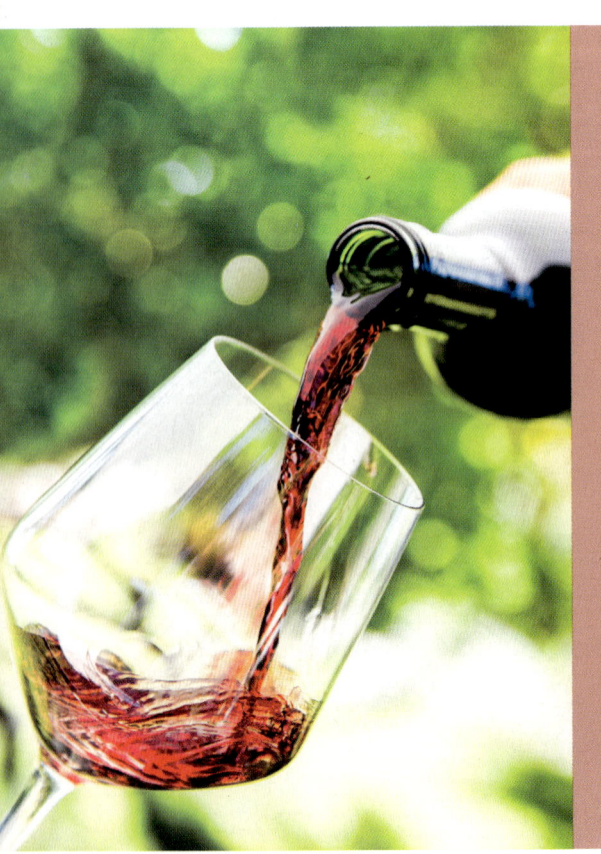

WHAT ABOUT HEALTH BENEFITS?

You might have heard that some alcohol is good for you – but is it true?

There are often news headlines touting the benefits of certain types of alcohol.

RED WINE IS PACKED WITH ANTIOXIDANTS THAT HELP THE HEART!

BEER CAN GIVE YOU STRONGER BONES!

DARK ALES HELP YOUR GUT MICROBIOME!

However, while there may be small benefits to some types of drink, the risks of drinking alcohol still outweigh any benefits. It's certainly not a reason to start drinking if you don't already. If you do drink, you may use this evidence to help choose what alcoholic drink to have, but it all applies in small quantities. If you're drinking a lot, there is likely to be no health benefits at all.

The best thing that you can do is choose a good-quality alcohol, drink under the recommended guidelines and consume plenty of water. This is how you can incorporate alcohol into a healthy, balanced lifestyle.

[1] Alcohol Intake and Blood Pressure Levels: A Dose-Response Meta-Analysis of Nonexperimental Cohort Studies, Hypertension Journal, 2023. [2] drinkaware.co.uk.

MANAGING ALCOHOL CONSUMPTION

AGE MATTERS
In the UK, the highest prevalence of drinking on at least one day each week is in adults aged 65 to 74 years.[2]

SEEK HELP WITH DRINKING

If you think you have a problem with alcohol, there is support out there for you

When you start to become more mindful of your alcohol intake, you could realise that you are drinking more than you should. You might need to seek extra support if you often feel the urge to have a drink, if others have mentioned your drinking to you, or if drinking alcohol leads to you making bad decisions or getting into difficult situations. You can visit your doctor to ask about help to quit drinking as a first port of call, or there are plenty of online resources, which can be good if you want advice on cutting down.

If you feel that you have become dependent on alcohol and can't give it up on your own, then there are alcohol addiction support groups, both online and in-person. It's usually better to get in-person support, as this gives you the accountability you need. If you are very dependent on alcohol, you may also have to go through the symptoms of alcohol withdrawal. Alcoholics Anonymous can be a good place to start for advice and resources: alcoholics-anonymous.org.uk or aa.org. Don't leave it too late to seek help and support.

CUTTING DOWN OR CUTTING IT OUT

It can be hard to consider cutting down on alcohol, particularly if it's a big part of your life currently. However, there are some tips you can try to help reduce your intake and bring down your blood pressure.

First you need to be honest about your current alcohol intake. This means knowing how many times a week you drink and how many units. As units can vary by alcohol type and from brand to brand, it can be useful to use a tracker to log all your drinking for a week – try to replicate a normal week for you. This will give you an idea of how many units you consume in a typical week. It might also give you some insight into how many excess calories you might be consuming through alcohol as well.

One way you can start to cut down without making any huge changes is to alter what you drink. You could look for lower-alcohol versions of your favourite drinks – one brand of wine can be very different to another, for example. You may also want to experiment with some of the many alcohol-free or low-alcohol brands on the market. You could alternate between an alcoholic drink and a non-alcoholic drink when you're out to reduce how much alcohol you consume. Other simple swaps to cut down include switching from large glasses of wine to smaller ones, adding soda water to wine to make it seem larger, picking single over double measures, and opting for bottles over pints. All of these will lower the volume of alcohol that you're drinking. When you are drinking, try to ensure that you're looking after other areas of your lifestyle. Eat a healthy, balanced meal before or with a drink, have plenty of water, and plan in alcohol-free days afterwards.

If you have been advised to give up completely, depending on the severity of your hypertension, you may find this hard. It can help if you have the support of friends and family, and you may want to avoid social situations where alcohol is expected for a short time while you get to grips with the change in your lifestyle.

Images Getty

MANAGING HYPERTENSION

SMOKING AND HYPERTENSION

Smoking is a risk factor for hypertension, and quitting has huge benefits for your health and heart

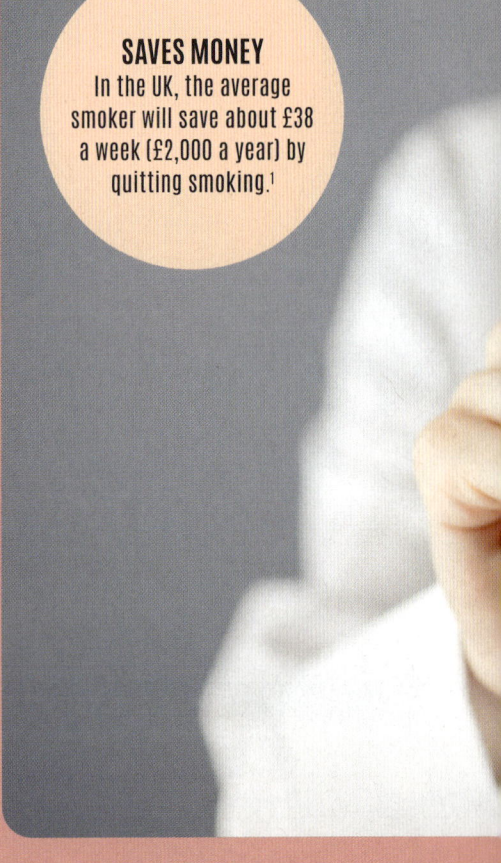

SAVES MONEY
In the UK, the average smoker will save about £38 a week (£2,000 a year) by quitting smoking.[1]

There is little doubt that smoking affects blood pressure. It is one of the biggest preventable risk factors for hypertension. Quitting smoking is one of the best things you can do for your overall health.

As well as increasing your blood pressure, smoking is the leading cause of cancer and cancer-related deaths. It can cause serious lung conditions like chronic obstructive pulmonary disease (COPD), obstructive sleep apnoea (which is also linked to hypertension), pneumonia and lung cancer. Because of the prevalence of hypertension among smokers, it also raises your risk of heart attacks and stroke. It can reduce your lifespan too – on average, you're likely to live ten years less than a non-smoker.

The danger lies in the tobacco, which contains more than 5,000 different chemicals that pollute the body every time you inhale. One of these is nicotine, which is an addictive substance. But the most harmful elements of tobacco are the tar, carbon monoxide and other chemicals in the smoke. This is why second-hand smoking is such a big problem – anyone around a smoker a lot is also at risk of health problems.

If you already have underlying conditions, smoking can make them worse. For example, those with asthma will need higher doses of steroids to manage the condition. If you have an existing lung condition, smoking can make it significantly worse and harder to control. It also impacts on your immune system, meaning that you're more likely to catch viruses than non-smokers.

The problem is that stopping smoking is difficult. The nicotine creates a powerful addiction, and you will feel intense urges to smoke. It can be really hard to combat these urges, especially when you have a strong daily routine built around smoking. Many people also use smoking to help cope with stress and anxiety, so taking away this coping mechanism means replacing it with another. Some people combine unhealthy habits, for example drinking alcohol and smoking – both of which are risk factors for hypertension, so the two together makes it even worse.

It doesn't matter whether you smoke rolled cigarettes or ready-made ones, low tar, light or menthol varieties, they will all contribute to poorer health outcomes.

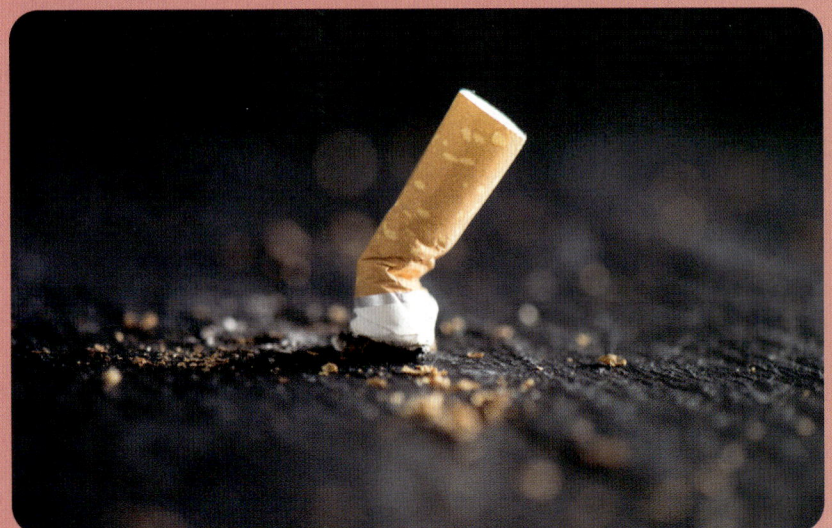

[1] NHS UK

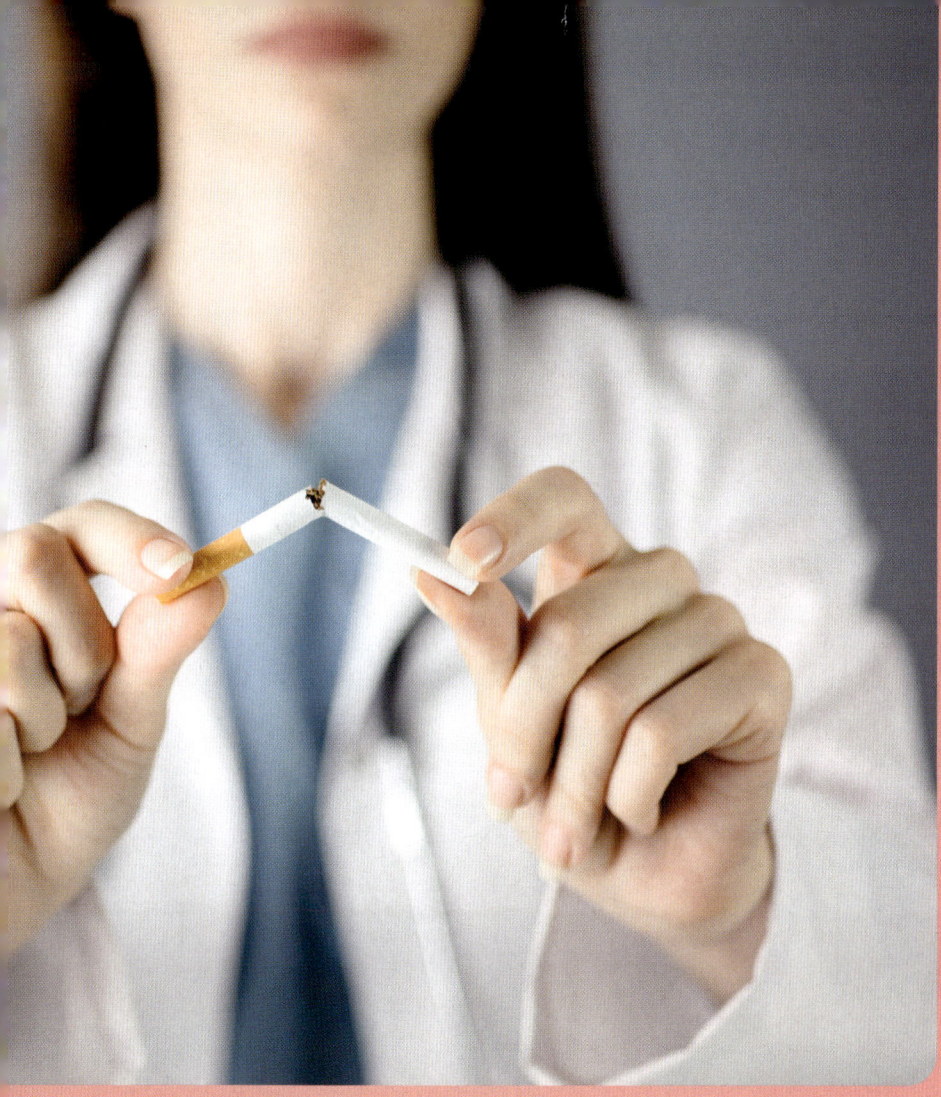

SMOKING AND HYPERTENSION

"IF YOU HAVE UNDERLYING CONDITIONS, SMOKING CAN MAKE THEM WORSE"

This is when fat deposits line the walls of your arteries, narrowing them. This can lead to your arteries becoming less flexible, making your blood more likely to clot, and forcing the heart to work harder than it usually does. Having high blood pressure on its own already causes the arteries to become narrower, so smoking when you have hypertension can exacerbate the process.

As the arteries get more clogged, your risk of having a serious heart attack or stroke gets higher. It also means that less oxygen can be carried around your body to other organs, which can lead to more damage.

What smoking does to blood pressure

Every time you light up a cigarette and inhale, your body experiences a temporary rise in blood pressure. This is due to the nicotine stimulating the hormones epinephrine and norepinephrine, which raise blood pressure. The nicotine also triggers the brain to release dopamine, which makes you feel good and is part of the reason that it becomes so addictive. You will also experience a rise in heart rate.

This rise in blood pressure (and heart rate) is short term, meaning that it should drop again within half an hour of finishing a cigarette. However, for people who smoke regularly, this short-term rise in blood pressure could be happening over and over again, meaning that they spend a lot of the day with elevated blood pressure. For someone who already has high blood pressure, these short-term rises can end up being more dangerous.

Over time, smoking starts to damage the walls of the blood vessels and increases the likelihood of developing atherosclerosis due to the sticky chemicals in the tobacco smoke.

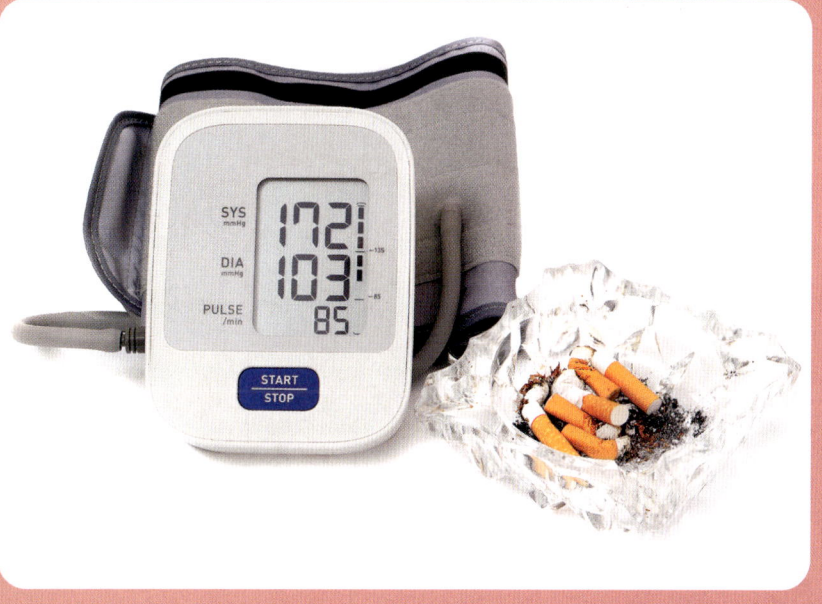

Image Getty

MANAGING
HYPERTENSION

Smoking makes it more likely that you will have other risk factors that contribute to hypertension. For example, people who smoke heavily may find it difficult to exercise due to problems with their lungs and breathing. Not getting enough physical activity can increase the risk of hypertension. Smoking can also lead to a loss of taste and smell, which can mean that you're more likely to have overly salty or sweet foods in order to deliver maximum flavour.

How to quit smoking

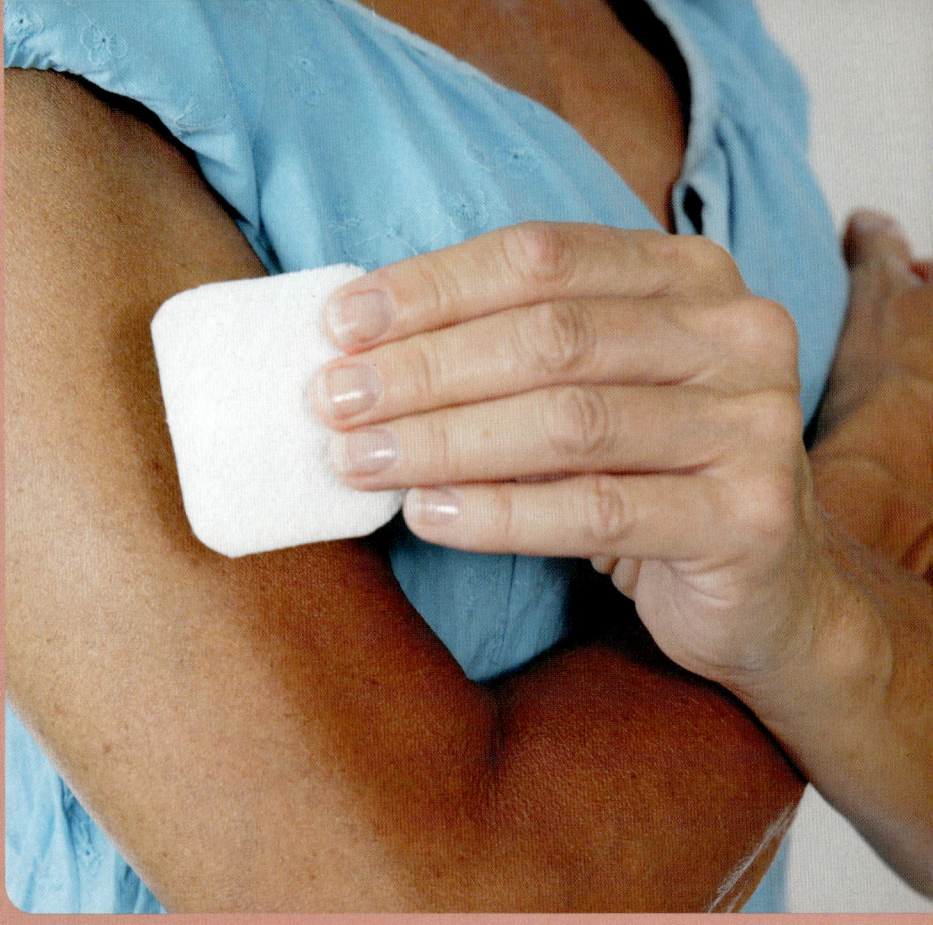

It is never too late to make the decision to stop smoking. The sooner you stop smoking, the better your outcome. According to the British Heart Foundation, if you quit smoking in your 30s, you could add an average of ten years to your life; if you quit at 60, you could add three more years to your life.

Unfortunately, it can be very difficult to break the habit, as well as combat the urge to smoke. It's well known that you're more likely to succeed if you have help to do so. There are many different programmes and services that are designed to help you stop smoking, including in-person groups, smoking advisors, online forums, apps and support services. You can go to your doctor in the first instance to be referred to local and online resources, as well as find out more about the products available that can help you to quit.

Products include items like e-cigarettes (see the box on page 73 on vaping), nicotine patches, nicotine gum and inhalers. These are designed to help you stop using cigarettes and the harmful tobacco, while helping with the nicotine addiction. Products like these can help you to quit, and

> "IT CAN BE VERY DIFFICULT TO BREAK THE HABIT, AS WELL AS COMBAT THE URGE TO SMOKE"

while you won't want to use them forever, they offer you a bridge to move on from smoking.

Group or individual support services can help you to put together an action plan, including why you want to stop smoking, and to set a date of when you'd like to be smoke-free. Usually, a treatment plan will include regular appointments, either in-person or over the phone, to help keep you on track, as well as a helpline to call if you're struggling with cravings. They can also help if you have a relapse and get you back where you want to be. If you don't have access to this kind of service, you could ask a friend or family member to be your accountability person, who you can call if you're finding it hard and who can remind you of why you wanted to quit in the first place.

There are also practical steps you can do while quitting. For example, when you get an intense craving, you need to do something to distract yourself while the craving passes. This can take between five and ten minutes, so maybe go for a walk or find something to do with your hands, such as a craft, jigsaw puzzle or game on your phone. You may have times of the day when you smoke that are hardwired into your brain, such as first thing in the morning or after a meal. It is hard to break these associations, but you can make new ones. Some people, for example, find it helps to brush their teeth after a meal when they would usually smoke, or go for a walk on their lunch break after eating.

The most important thing is to keep going – if you have a bad day or even if you do have a cigarette, every time you choose not to smoke is a step in the right direction for your health and your blood pressure.

SMOKING AND HYPERTENSION

WHAT HAPPENS WHEN YOU STOP SMOKING

Trace the timeline of recovery when you stop using cigarettes

You might think that it's too late and the damage is done if you've been a smoker for a long time, but your body can recover quite quickly from some of the health issues related to smoking. Here is a timeline of some of the biggest changes you can experience:

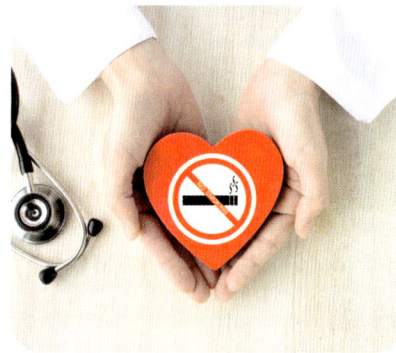

First 20-30 minutes
Your blood pressure and heart rate drop from the spike caused by inhaling nicotine.

2-3 days
The carbon monoxide levels in your body return to normal.

2 weeks
Circulation and lung function start to improve.

First year
You should be able to breathe more deeply, with less shortness of breath. You should also notice that you're coughing less, but when you do cough it's more productive, helping to clear the lungs.

3-6 years
The risk of coronary heart disease is reduced by 50%.

5-10 years
The risk of cancer of the mouth, throat and voice box is halved, and the risk of stroke decreases.

After 10 years
The risk of lung cancer is reduced by 50%. The risk of other cancers (bladder, oesophagus and kidneys) decreases.

After 15 years
The risk of coronary heart disease is almost the same as a non-smoker.

WHAT ABOUT VAPING?

A quick look at whether vaping has an impact on blood pressure

The use of e-cigarettes, or vapes, has risen rapidly over the last few years. They offer a nicotine hit but without the tobacco, and they can be flavoured to make them more palatable. They can be a useful tool for those who are trying to quit smoking. One small study from the University of Dundee (2019) found that within a month of swapping from tobacco to e-cigarettes blood vessel health, including blood pressure, started to improve.

However, this is not the same as saying they're safe, as they're too new to have any long-term data on how they impact blood pressure and heart health. There was a 2023 study[2] that interpreted the results of its data saying: 'ENDS [electronic nicotine delivery systems] users had acute worsening of blood pressure, heart rate, and heart rate variability… after vaping, compared to control participants'.

Ideally, vapes should only be used by those trying to give up tobacco, with the ultimate aim of stopping use over time.

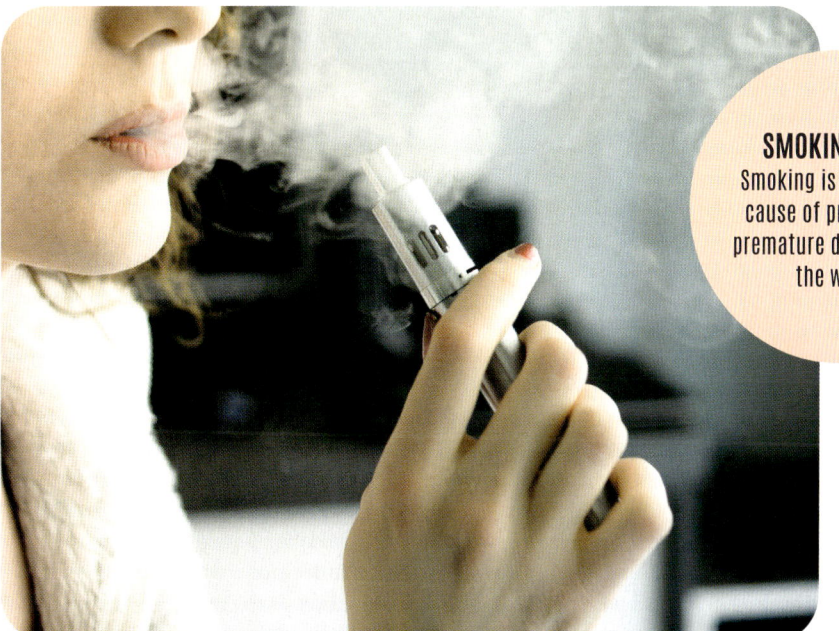

SMOKING KILLS
Smoking is the leading cause of preventable, premature death around the world.

[1] American Heart Association. [2] Cardiovascular and Pulmonary Responses to Acute Use of Electronic Nicotine Delivery Systems and Combustible Cigarettes in Long-Term Users, CHEST, September 2023.

MANAGING
HYPERTENSION

SUPPORT GROUPS AND RESOURCES

Where to turn for extra blood pressure help, support and advice

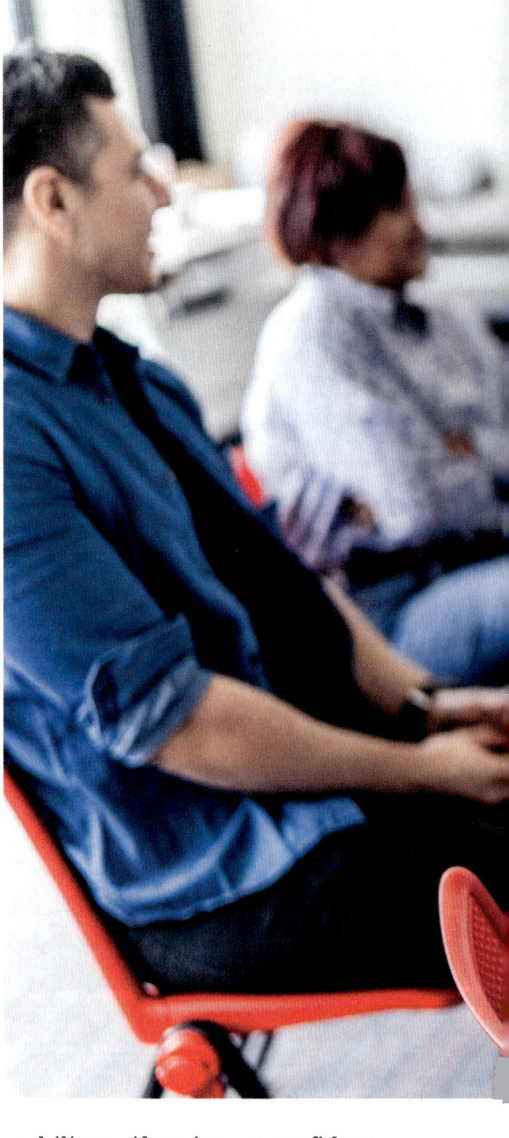

If you're struggling to come to terms with having hypertension, the medication, or making the necessary lifestyle changes, you may benefit from finding support groups or using online resources. Groups, forums and helplines are good for answering any specific questions you have and for getting advice, but for many people, the biggest benefit is that they feel less alone. Other people in the same situation will understand what you're going through, and may share the same goals or have similar health complications.

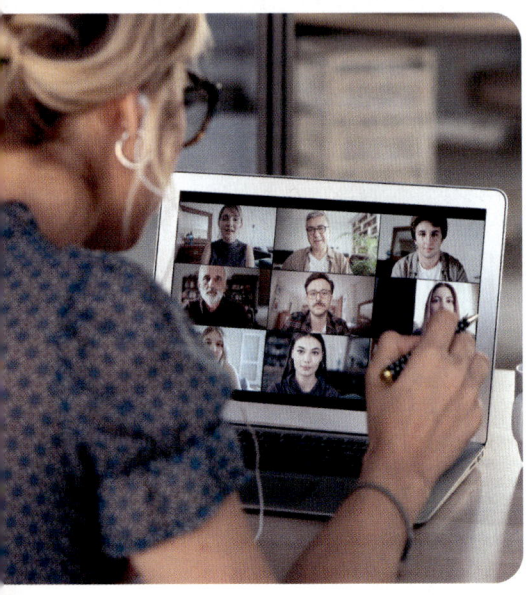

In the first instance, you may find it helpful to speak to your doctor or nurse to see if they can advise of any suitable support groups in your local area. They may be able to refer you directly or give you advice on how to self-refer. These in-person groups are a good way to meet new people and talk about what you're experiencing in a safe and private environment. The groups might be specifically for those with hypertension, or they may be focused on a certain health issue that can be caused by high blood pressure. For example, in the UK, the British Heart Foundation has more than 120 affiliated Heart Support Groups for people affected by heart and circulatory diseases. There are also groups for younger people with hypertension, groups that focus on physical activity, and groups that educate about nutrition and weight loss. If you have an additional health condition, like diabetes, or are going through a life stage, like menopause, then there are groups available for these, where you may also meet people with high blood pressure.

Of course, you might prefer to find online support. This can be a good option for those with limited mobility or if you're not confident with in-person sessions. Support ranges from courses and webinars that you can attend to learn more about managing hypertension, to forums where you can chat with like-minded people. Again, speaking to your medical team is a good place to start, as they can often point you to different resources online.

If you have a specific question or concern about your blood pressure, your own doctor is usually the first port of call. But we know that medical services can sometimes be a bit stretched and you may need to get advice from elsewhere. There are quite a few helplines set up to answer your questions and point you in the right direction. Otherwise, there

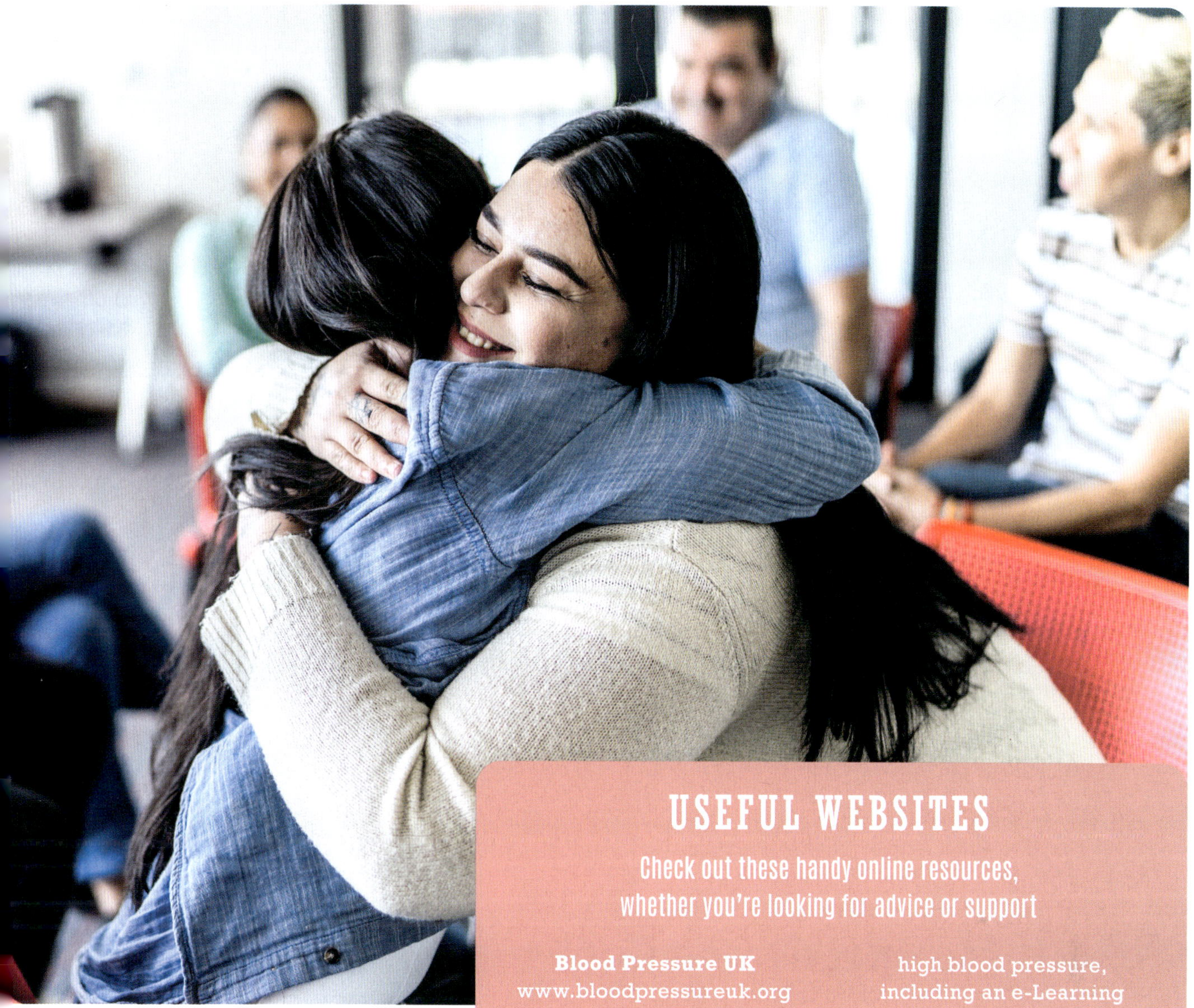

SUPPORT GROUPS AND RESOURCES

are some great websites (see the box to the right) that you can visit to start educating yourself about the latest guidelines, treatments and news to help you understand your condition and how to treat it.

Don't be afraid to reach out in real life, too. You might be surprised by how many people in your life have been impacted by hypertension – sometimes it just takes one person to start a conversation. Even if your friendship circle or family aren't able to give you advice on high blood pressure, you can get them involved in your treatment plan. For example, if you are trying to lose weight, improve your diet or get more exercise, having company and support for this will make it far easier.

USEFUL WEBSITES

Check out these handy online resources, whether you're looking for advice or support

Blood Pressure UK
www.bloodpressureuk.org
A charity dedicated to lowering blood pressure, this website is full of useful guides, has a helpline to ask any questions about hypertension, and has a really useful learning centre.

British Heart Foundation
www.bhf.org.uk
Written and audio guides to high blood pressure, as well as handy videos on key topics, links to support groups – both in person and online – and a helpline to get advice.

American Heart Association
www.heart.org
Lots of resources looking at high blood pressure, including an e-Learning module, a guide for talking to a healthcare professional, fact sheets and a support network.

Patients Like Me
www.patientslikeme.com
The world's largest patient community where you can directly speak to thousands of people worldwide with the same condition or conditions.

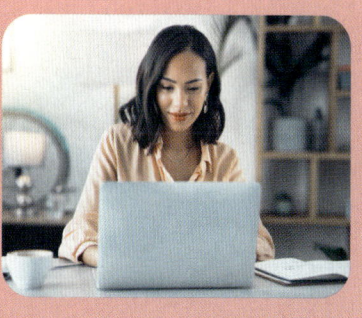

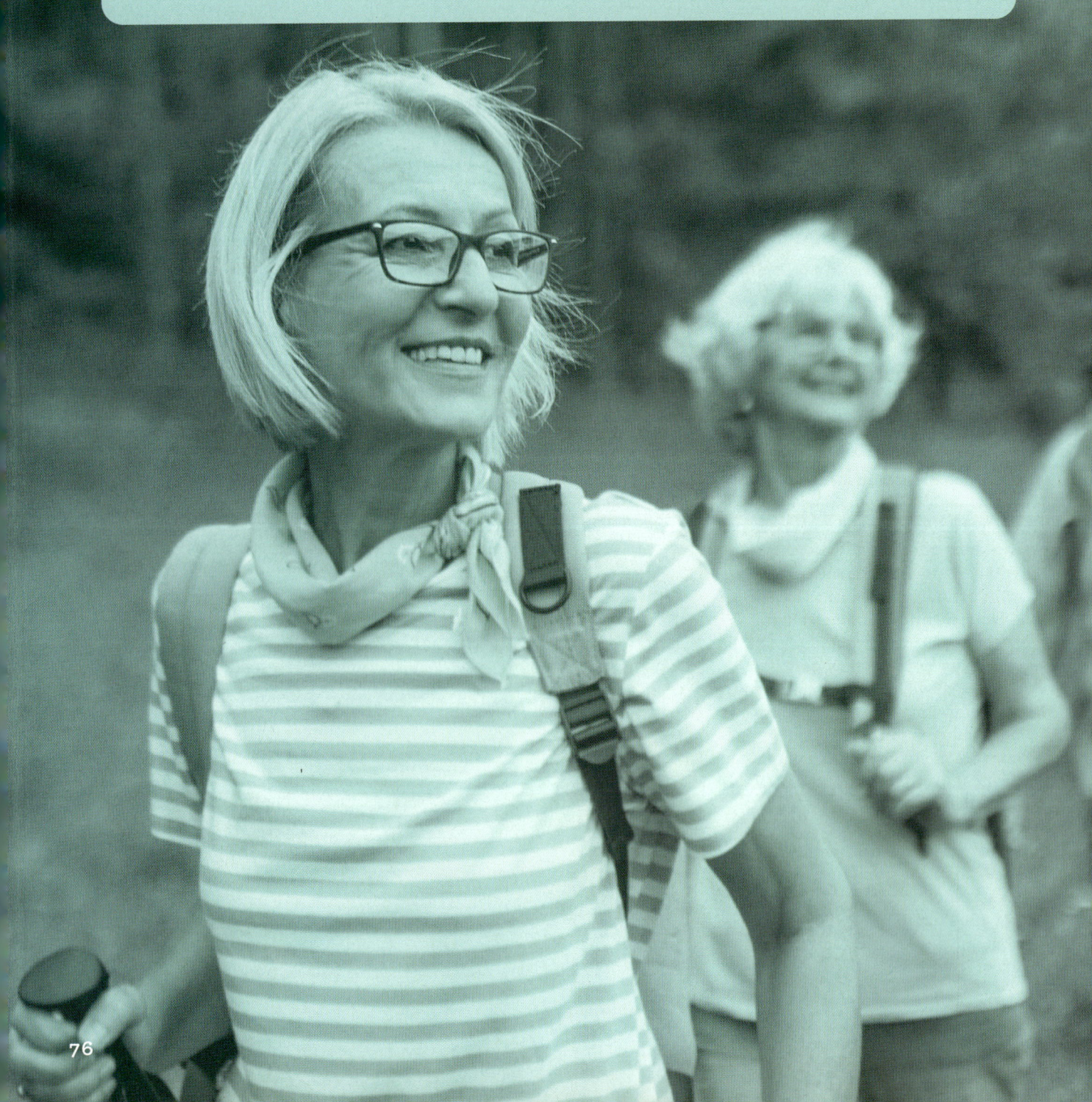

LIFESTYLE

Discover the importance of maintaining a healthy diet, exercising regularly, prioritising sleep and much more

3

78
OPTIMISE YOUR LIFESTYLE

82
THE IMPORTANCE OF PHYSICAL ACTIVITY

88
THE BEST TYPES OF EXERCISE FOR HYPERTENSION

92
IMPROVE YOUR SLEEP

96
HOW TO EAT FOR HYPERTENSION

102
TOP 10 FOODS FOR HYPERTENSION

LIFESTYLE

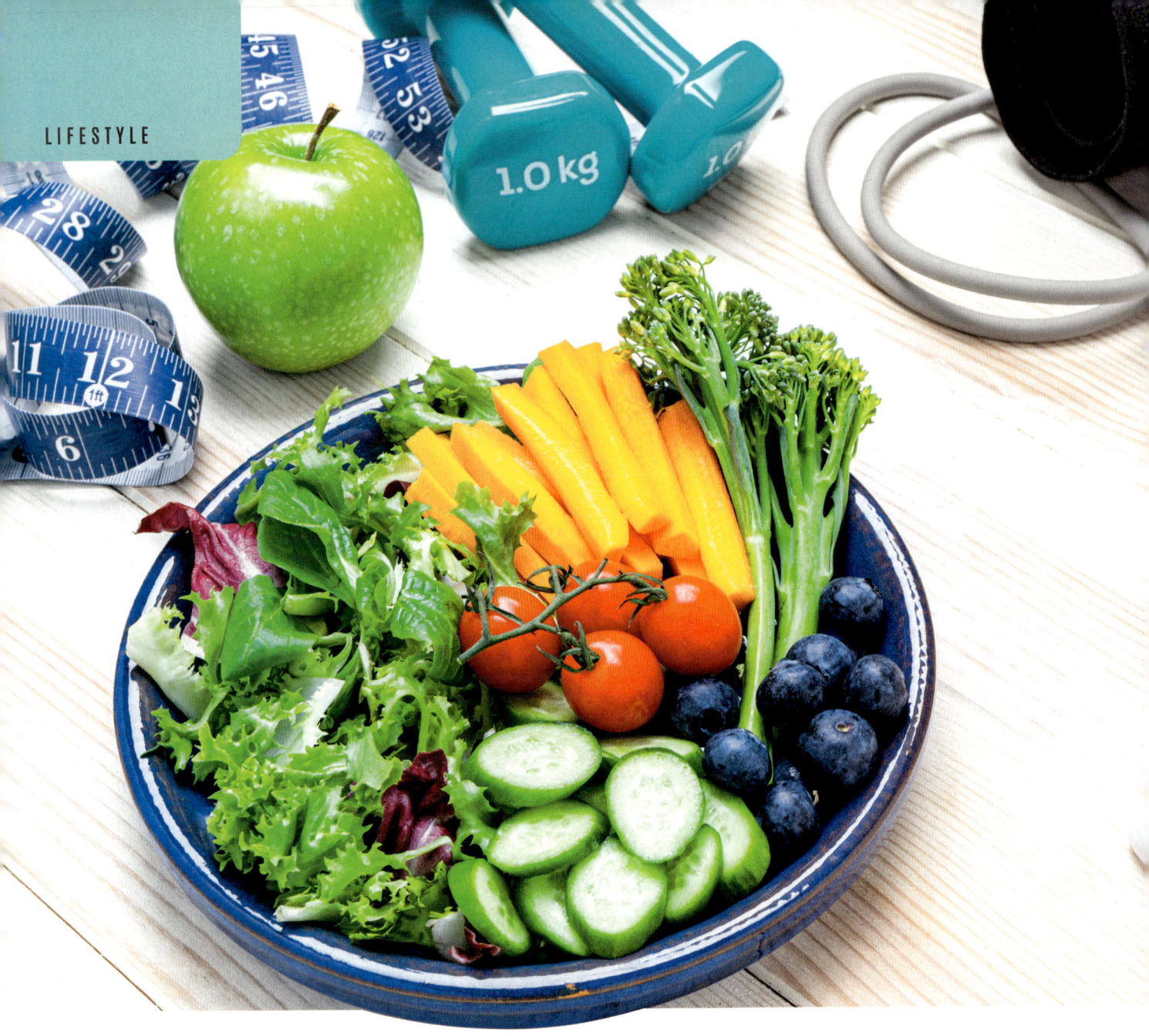

OPTIMISE YOUR LIFESTYLE

The life choices you make every day can impact on how quickly you get your blood pressure under control

Getting your blood pressure under control and maintaining it means working towards a healthy lifestyle. This might be in conjunction with other treatment plans, such as medication, stopping smoking, cutting down on alcohol, losing weight and lowering your stress levels.

In fact, a healthy lifestyle will help with all of those too! It can make any medicines you're taking work most effectively and can contribute to weight management, good sleep and a calmer mind. You might need to work on other areas of your treatment plan first, before tackling lifestyle interventions. For example, you may need to let your medicines start to work before you make

OPTIMISE YOUR LIFESTYLE

THE WHOLE-BODY APPROACH

When it comes to lifestyle changes, the holistic approach works best. Everything is interconnected and by working on one area, others will benefit too. So, when you work on getting good-quality sleep, this will have a knock-on effect on your physical activity levels, energy and focus. When you're more active, you get better sleep, make better food choices and improve your self-esteem. Following a healthy and balanced diet gives you more fuel for exercise, improves your mental health, and helps you to cope better with stress. Lifestyle changes all work together.

That doesn't mean that you have to do everything all at once. You may decide to focus on one single area to start off with, or you may prefer to do one little thing in each of the different lifestyle areas. There is often a snowball effect of healthy habits – once you start doing a few things better than before, it can give you the focus and motivation to make further changes in other areas.

When you're told that you need to make lifestyle changes to improve your health, it can sometimes feel like a punishment – giving up the food you love and the drinks you want, and having to do more exercise than you would like. However, you can find a way to keep doing everything you want with some small changes. Try not to focus on what you can or can't do or have. Try instead to think about what making changes will give you: a healthier, happier you.

This is about taking back control of your health – we can sometimes feel like it's too late or too hard to make changes, but that's not true. You can make the decision to build a lifestyle that works for you and your future health at any time.

THINK LIFELONG
Lifestyle interventions aren't short-term fixes; you need to make changes that will stay with you forever.

too many other changes, or you might need to look at getting your weight under control before considering exercise.

However, you can set lifestyle goals a little at a time. This section of this bookazine will go through what it means to live a healthy lifestyle and how that benefits your blood pressure, but feel free to dip in and out of the pages depending on your goals.

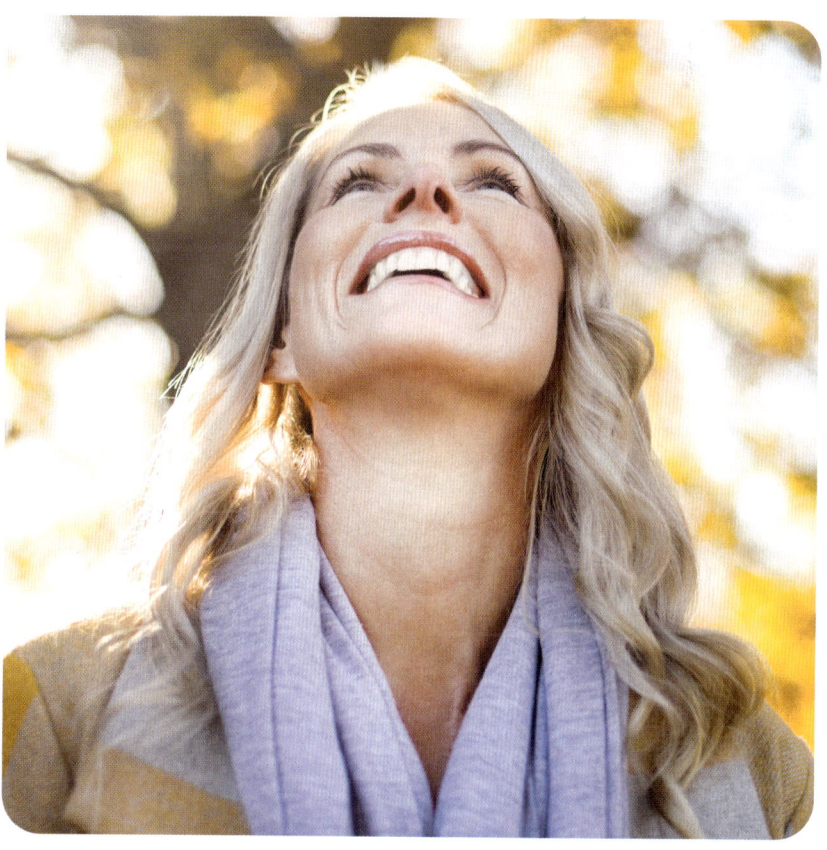

Images Getty

79

LIFESTYLE

THE SECRET TO LIFESTYLE SUCCESS

Making lifestyle changes stick is the hardest part. You can be very motivated at first, but as time goes on, it can be harder to stay on track, especially if the results you want are taking time to appear.

It can help if you have a good support network around you. Doing things alone takes more willpower and can feel very isolated. If you have family close by, ask them to support you in your journey towards a healthier lifestyle. It can benefit everyone, especially if you all contribute towards ideas for a meal plan or go for walks together, for example. Sometimes you might need to lean on friends, who can give you a boost when you're finding it hard. If you don't have anyone close to you who you can rely on to give you the support you need, then have a look for local community groups, gyms, wellbeing centres and clubs where you can be around likeminded people to help you with your progress.

Another way to be successful in making lifestyle changes is to make sure that you're setting clear goals. We often talk about the SMART system of goal setting, as this helps you to make goals that you're more likely to keep. SMART goals are ones that are very specific and things you can measure. A good example is if you're trying to cut down on alcohol, for example. 'Cutting down on alcohol' is a very vague sentence – what does that mean? You can set a goal that you'd like to ensure you have no more than 14 units a week (the recommended limit) with at least three days a week where you drink no alcohol. This is very 'specific' and it's also easy to keep track of. A SMART goal also needs to be 'achievable' – so, for example, dropping to 14 units a week might be more achievable than going to nothing at all straight away. Your goals should be 'relevant' – ie they have a purpose that you're dedicated to achieving. Finally, your goal should be 'time-bound', so don't forget to set a deadline in which to achieve your goal.

Write your goals down and make sure they are somewhere you can see them. If you have quite big overall goals, you can break them down and set smaller goals along the way to keep you motivated. You may also like to set rewards for each milestone you get to. Try not to make these rewards something that you're actively working to avoid in your new lifestyle, ie if you're changing your diet, you don't really want to use something like chocolate as a reward. Instead, why not pick something that makes you feel happy, such as a new book or going to watch a movie.

"MAKE SURE THAT YOU'RE SETTING CLEAR GOALS"

COPING WITH BAD DAYS
What to do when mistakes happen, and how to learn from them and get back on track

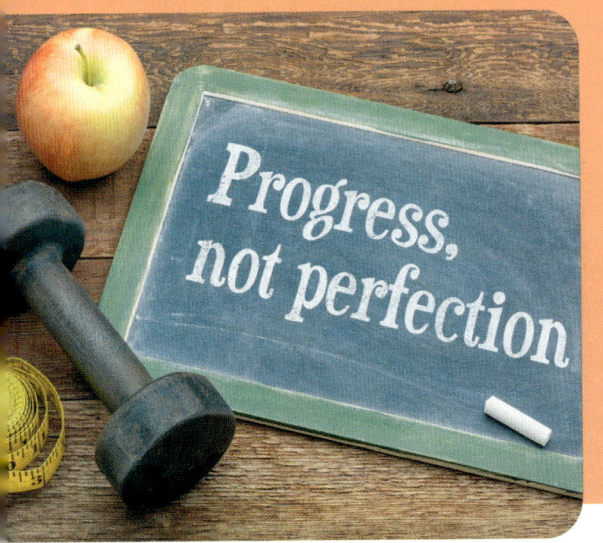

No matter how invested you are in a healthy lifestyle, you will have bad days. You will reach for the junk food, skip a workout or have too much to drink. None of us are perfect, and we all have days when we make choices that are less than optimal. And that's okay!

We're aiming for progress and not perfection. One bad day won't impact on your end results, as long as one bad day doesn't turn into a bad week, month or year. When you've had a bad day, first you need to accept it and let it go. It's in the past now and your decisions about today are all that matter. Try to look at what triggered the bad day – was it a stressful time at work or did you sleep badly? This can help you learn what you could do differently if faced with the same situation again. Reset your mindset and carry on with your goals. The bumps in the road are all part of the journey.

OPTIMISE YOUR LIFESTYLE

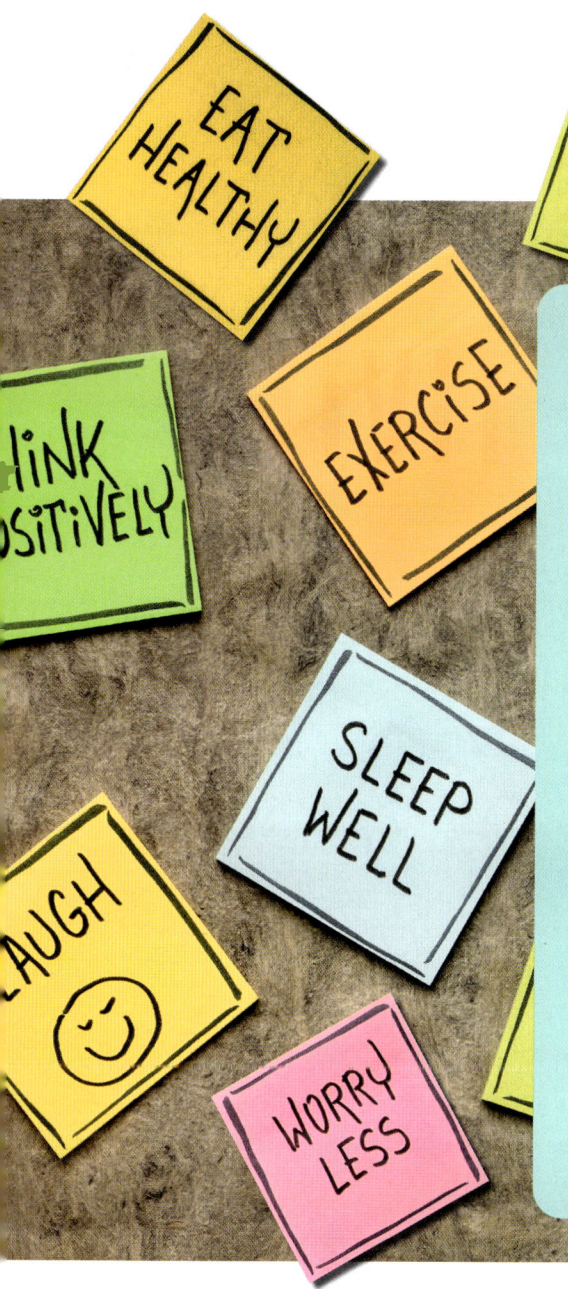

REMEMBER YOUR 'WHY'

Having a clear reason for wanting to make changes can help you to stay motivated

When you're making big changes to your lifestyle, especially if you're looking to make a lot of changes in many different areas of your life, it can feel really hard to stay on track. Old habits are always easier to fall back into and you will be drawn to them. That's why you need to have a good reason to keep going and remind yourself of this from time to time, especially when it gets hard. Why do you want to reduce your blood pressure right now? Is it so you can be healthy for a long time for your children, or do you want to be able to go on certain adventures? Do you want to be more energetic, fitter and happier? Some people find it helpful to have a motivation board with photos or quotes on to act as a visual cue when you need a boost, or you could ask a loved one to support you on the journey and help you stay focused on your 'why'.

SHARE YOUR KNOWLEDGE
As you learn more about a healthy lifestyle, you can pass on your knowledge to others who might need some help.

BENEFITS OF A HEALTHY LIFESTYLE

There are so many benefits to living a healthy lifestyle and these go far beyond hypertension. Yes, making lifestyle changes will help with reducing your blood pressure and this is probably the trigger for you starting in the first place, but once you get started, you will be making your life better in so many other ways.

Not only will you improve your chances of living longer, but you'll be living well in that time too. If you are eating well and doing exercise, you will stay stronger as you age. This means you will be able to keep doing everything you love for as long as possible. This also gives you more time with your family and the ability to do more things with them, such as running around with a football, going on long hikes and even trying out some adventurous challenges!

When you're looking after yourself, this has a great effect on your mental wellbeing too. You might find that your self-esteem and self-confidence are greatly improved, and you may also feel happier, calmer and more stable in your moods. You may also find that you can cope with stress better and that you're more resilient. This can help to strengthen your relationships with other people too.

While thinking about how to get started might feel a bit overwhelming at first, when you start to explore all the possibilities ahead of you, you might even find that you start to feel a little excited. You are in charge of your own health and wellbeing, and when you make changes to your lifestyle, you will feel the benefits in your mind, body and soul.

LIFESTYLE

THE IMPORTANCE OF PHYSICAL ACTIVITY

Being more active is one of the best things you can do to reduce and manage your blood pressure

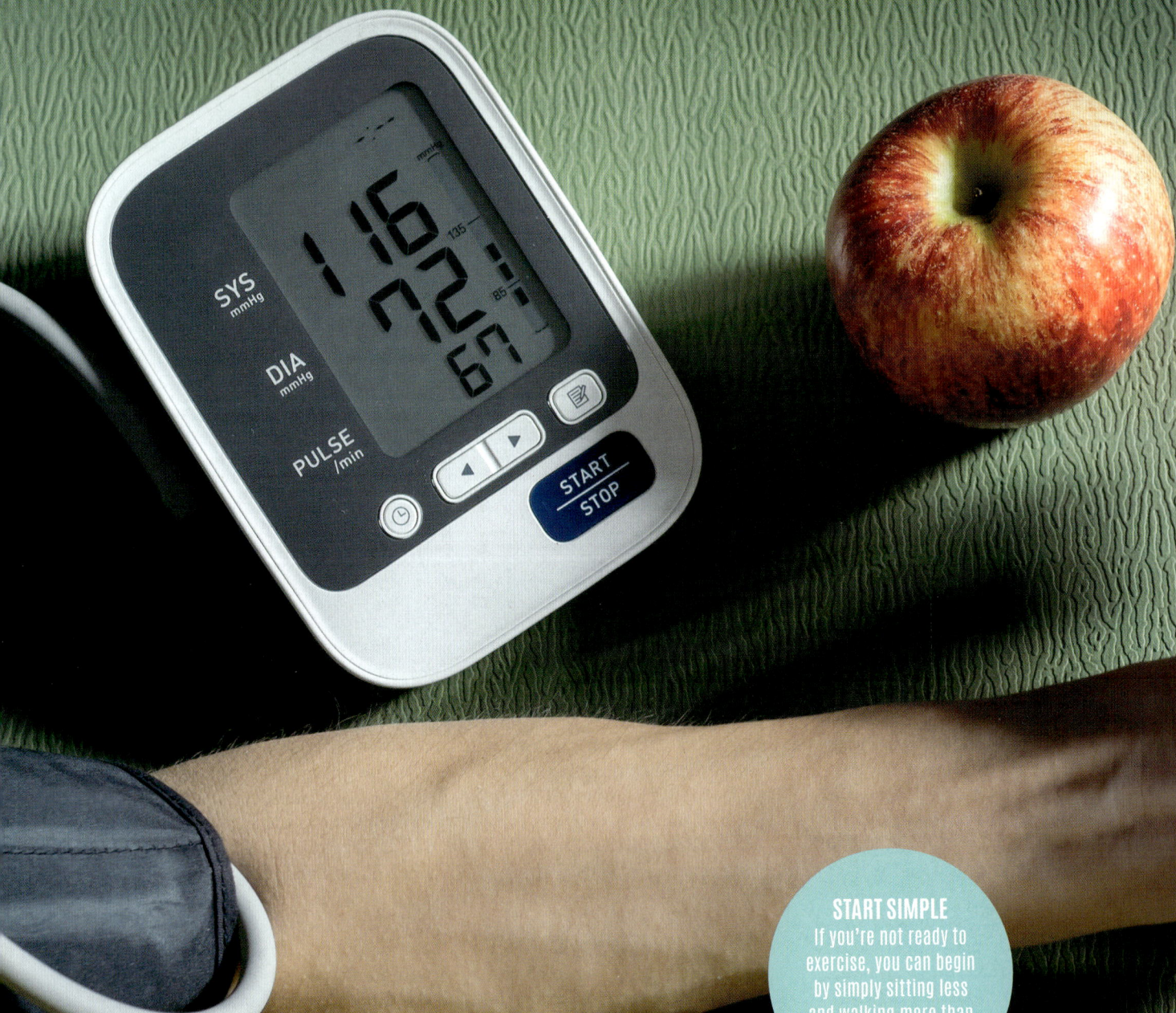

START SIMPLE
If you're not ready to exercise, you can begin by simply sitting less and walking more than you do now.

THE IMPORTANCE OF PHYSICAL ACTIVITY

HOW EXERCISE IMPACTS BLOOD PRESSURE

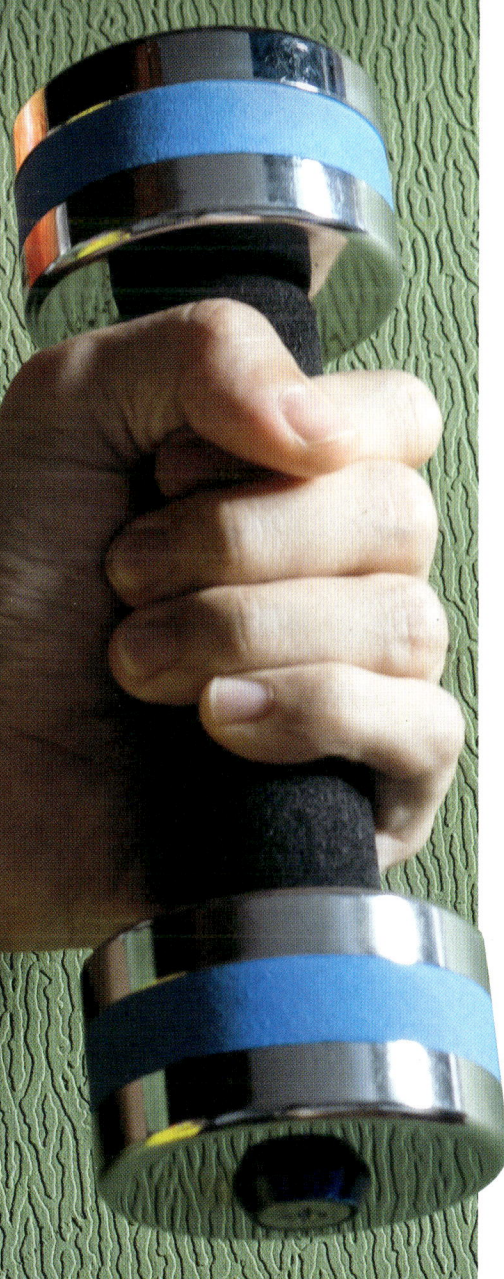

When you're diagnosed with hypertension, one of the primary treatments to help improve your blood pressure, as well as your cardiovascular health, is to get regular physical activity. It's an essential component of living a healthy lifestyle and if you're only making one change to your way of life, then making sure that you're moving enough every day should be it.

It doesn't mean you have to be running marathons or going to the gym day in and day out; regular physical activity is just that – moving your body on a regular basis every day in a way that suits you.

When you are active, your heart rate rises, and your heart has to pump harder. Doing this over and over again helps to strengthen your heart – it is a muscle like any other and benefits from being exercised. If you can build a strong, powerful heart, it can pump the blood around your body with less effort, reducing the pressure in your blood vessels and bringing your readings down.

There is a lot of research that backs up the fact that regular exercise lowers blood pressure, and this can start to happen quite quickly, usually within a few months. Regular activity can help to bring down both the diastolic and systolic readings, improving your overall health and reducing your risk of the complications associated with hypertension, like heart disease, heart attacks and strokes. When you exercise, it also helps to improve blood flow to your muscles and organs, which can help them to work optimally; your blood vessels become more relaxed, enabling your blood to flow more freely; and you release excess salt from the body in your sweat, which can also help to lower blood pressure.

Regular physical activity also helps you to manage other risk factors for hypertension. If you need to lose weight to get to a healthy level, then exercising alongside a balanced diet can help you to see results. It also helps you to get plenty of high-quality sleep, which can have a positive effect on your blood pressure, as can reducing your levels of long-term stress. Those who exercise regularly may also be more inclined to eat nutritious food, which is a key factor in controlling your blood pressure. Combining blood pressure medication with exercise can help you to see a greater reduction in blood pressure than either of them alone – though you do need to check if there are any limitations when it comes to exercise related to your individual treatment plan.

One thing to bear in mind is that you need to keep doing regular physical activity to retain the benefits. The positive effect on your blood pressure continues as long as you do. If you stop exercising and become more sedentary, your blood pressure can start to rise again.

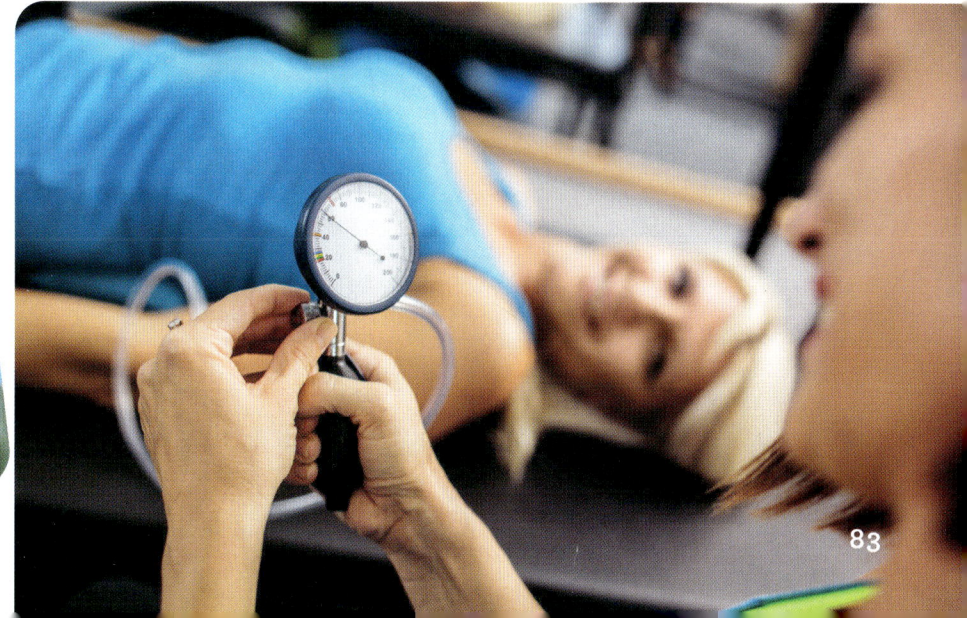

Images Getty

LIFESTYLE

BENEFITS OF BEING PHYSICALLY ACTIVE

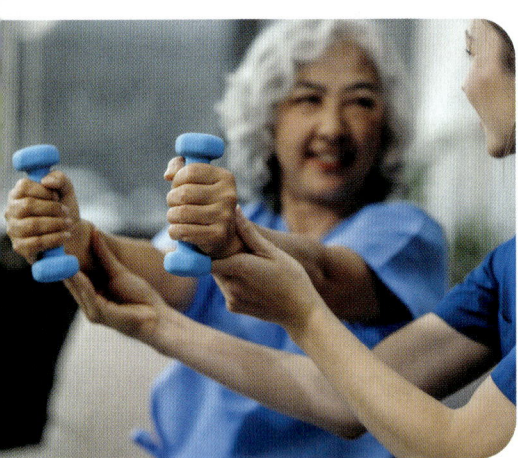

There are so many benefits to being physically active. We've already mentioned the significant impact that it has on your blood pressure, which is likely your primary reason for reading this book. However, being active has so many other benefits that will improve your quality of life, and your overall health and wellbeing.

Doing enough exercise helps to protect your heart, meaning that your risk of heart-related conditions is lower. It also improves and retains your lung health, which means that you can breathe deeply and take in enough oxygen. There are plenty of studies to show that being active can help to reduce your risk of certain cancers and type 2 diabetes. By building up your strength, it lowers your risk of bone disease, such as osteoporosis, and of falls in later life. In fact, physical activity helps to reduce the risk of all-cause mortality, according to the World Health Organization.

There are positive benefits for your mind too. Being active helps to reduce the risk of mental health conditions like anxiety and depression. It can help your cognition, by improving your memory and problem-solving skills, and enabling you to stay more focused and alert. The more you move your body now, the better it will move as you age, with strong muscles and flexible joints.

The human body is not designed to stay still, but in the modern world it's all too easy to sit for long periods of time. But if we want our body to function optimally, we need to use it as much as possible, every day. All the benefits you will experience will help you to control your hypertension and even start to reverse it.

FITNESS TRACKER
A basic wearable tracker can be helpful for seeing your progress and monitoring your overall wellbeing.

MAKE YOUR DAY-TO-DAY MORE ACTIVE

Work small bursts of activity into your normal life for maximum effect

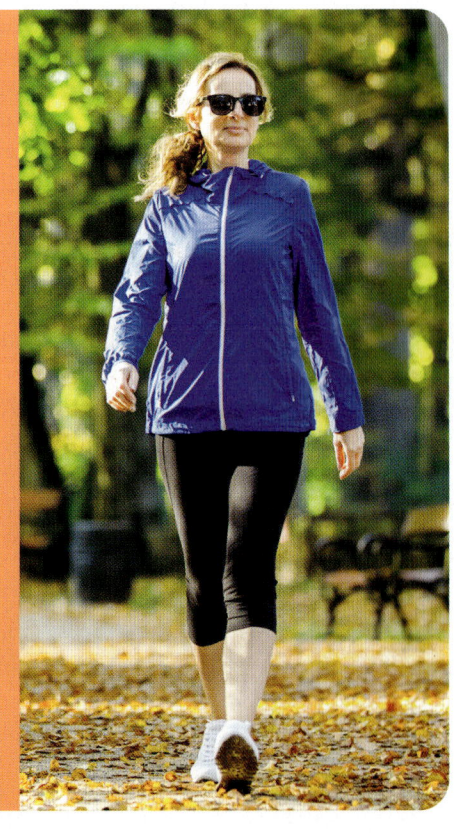

For some people, the thought of having to do formal 'exercise' can be quite overwhelming, or you might not have the time right now to dedicate to going to the gym or doing a home workout. However, you can get plenty of benefits from simply making your everyday life more active.

If you're sat down a lot at a sedentary job, and you commute by car or bus, then you may not be moving very much at all. It can take a little effort to find ways to become more active, but even the simplest changes will build up. If you can, try to make your commute more active by walking or cycling some of your journey, and ditch the car for short trips to the shops. Choose to take the stairs when you can.

Make sure that you have activity breaks during your day, even if it's just a few minutes of standing up, walking or stretching. Try to use your lunch break to get out for a walk if that's possible, or even consider seeing if you can get a standing desk if you spend a lot of time at a computer.

IS IT SAFE TO EXERCISE WITH HYPERTENSION?

If you have very high blood pressure, you may have to be more careful with exercise

Most people can exercise safely with hypertension and will be encouraged to. Your doctor should be able to advise you on ways to get started. If you've never exercised before, you may need to build up slowly in terms of both intensity and duration. However, if you have very high blood pressure you may be advised to follow a specific exercise programme or not start exercise until your blood pressure is more controlled. Because exercise causes a short-term rise in blood pressure – which usually drops quickly afterwards – this can be more of a worry for those with severe hypertension. You may need to focus on getting the right medication and other lifestyle interventions, like diet, first.

This table gives a general overview of whether it's safe to exercise with your blood pressure levels

Blood pressure readings	Can I exercise?
140/90mmHg – 179/99mmHg	If you fall into this high blood pressure range, you should be able to safely be more active in order to bring your readings down.
180/100mmHg – 199/109mmHg	As this is considered a very high reading, you should speak to your medical team before starting any new activity, but should generally be able to exercise and be more active.
200/110mmHg or higher	If you have severe hypertension, you should not start any new activity and urgently speak to your medical team.

HOW TO EXERCISE FOR HYPERTENSION

In general, a person with high blood pressure should be aiming for the same recommended minimum levels of activity as the general population. These guidelines are set out by the World Health Organization and have been adopted as national guidance by most countries' governing bodies.

Each week, physically capable adults should aim to do:

At least 150 minutes of moderate-intensity aerobic activity or 75 minutes of vigorous-intensity aerobic activity

Muscle-strengthening activities on two days or more

This equates to about 30 minutes a day for five days a week of moderate activity. For even more health benefits, adults can aim for at least 300 minutes of moderate-intensity aerobic activity or 150 minutes of vigorous-intensity aerobic activity (or a combination of both intensity levels).

On top of this intentional activity, you should also be looking at being less sedentary throughout the day. This means sitting down for less of the day, as we know that sitting too much is linked to poorer health outcomes. Of course, if you have an office job with long hours, it's not that easy. All we can do is maximise the time outside of the office. You should also try to take a five-minute break every hour to stand up and move around – you could set a reminder to do this to get in the habit. It's so easy to go from a long day sitting to wanting to wind down in front of the television or to read a book, for example, which means more sitting, so becoming more active can mean having to make quite a big lifestyle change.

For those with hypertension, making activity a priority is a must. It's so important if you need to get your readings to come down. Every little bit really does help. Multiple mini movement opportunities throughout the day start to add up. If you're currently not very active, then start small and build up. If you already exercise and have been diagnosed with high blood pressure, then you may want to focus first on being more active outside of your planned exercise schedule.

LIFESTYLE

WHAT EXERCISE TO DO (OR NOT DO)

When you start to exercise, either from scratch or with the intention to increase what you already do, then there are a few considerations to bear in mind if you're someone with high blood pressure. If you have very high blood pressure – severe hypertension – you should check with your doctor as to whether there are any limitations to what you can do, and get their advice before beginning a new exercise routine. There's more information about exercising safely with hypertension in the box on page 87.

You also need to check with your team if you have any other health conditions, for example, high cholesterol, a previous heart attack, a family history of heart problems or stroke, diabetes, lung disease or kidney disease, or if you're on prescribed medication. There will always be a way to be active, as physical activity can help with your overall health, but there may be certain types of exercise that you need to avoid.

For example, for people with hypertension, you may need to avoid extreme sports, especially if your blood pressure is not under control. So, if you're planning on doing anything like scuba diving or jumping out of a plane, you will need to see a doctor beforehand and see whether this is appropriate for you. Anything that can rapidly raise your blood pressure can be more dangerous for those who already have hypertension – even going on a theme park ride!

You may be advised to avoid certain types of exercise that also cause a rapid rise in blood pressure, such as sprinting fast, playing squash or weightlifting. However, most exercise types will be appropriate, including walking, cycling, rowing, dancing, running, tennis and gardening.

If you have mobility problems, you can try some chair-based exercise to help boost your activity levels. You can do this yourself, under the guidance of an exercise professional, by following an online course, or by attending an in-person class. Chair-based activity works on building your strength and flexibility, as well as working your heart, but without putting strain on your lower body.

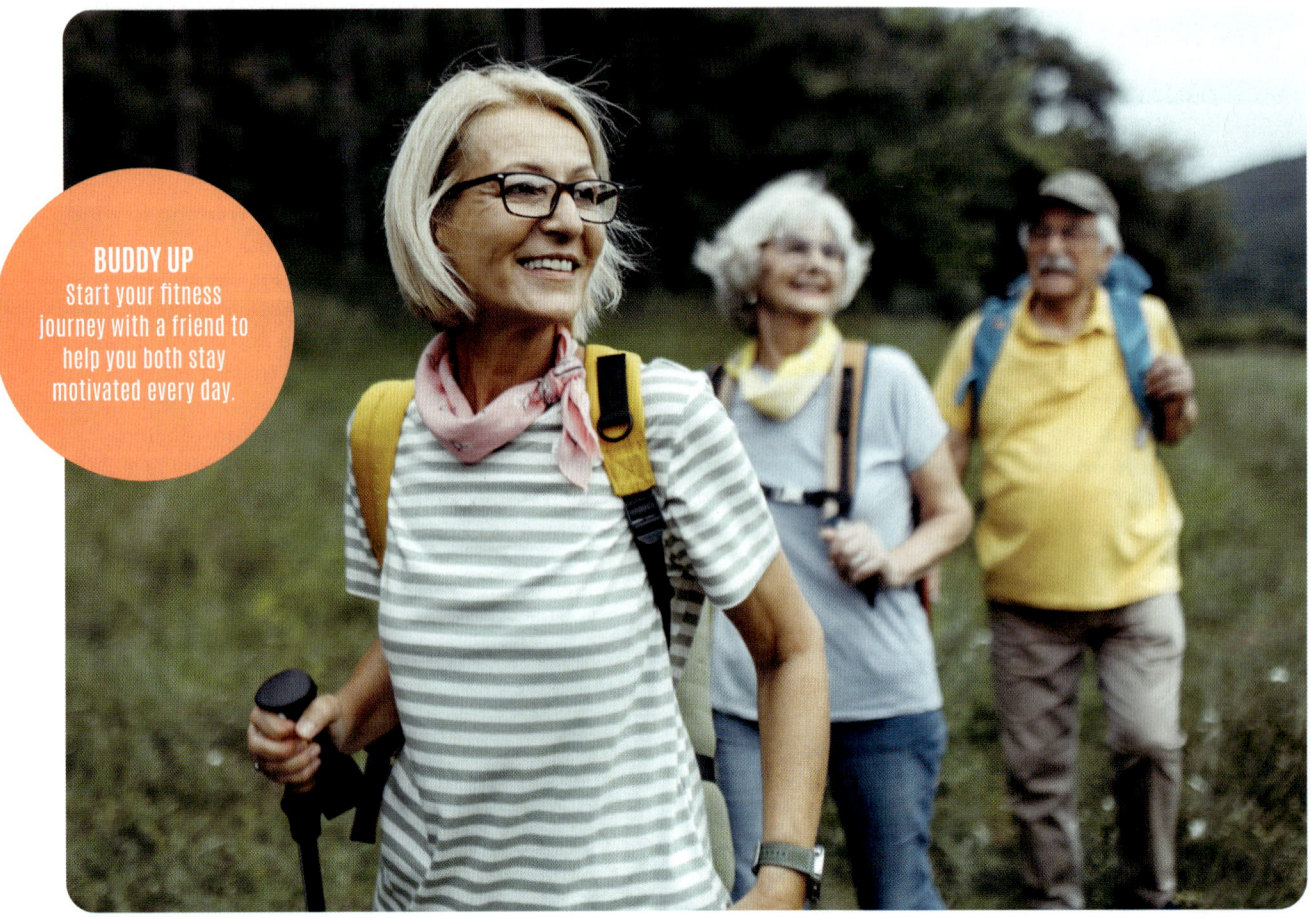

BUDDY UP
Start your fitness journey with a friend to help you both stay motivated every day.

THE IMPORTANCE OF PHYSICAL ACTIVITY

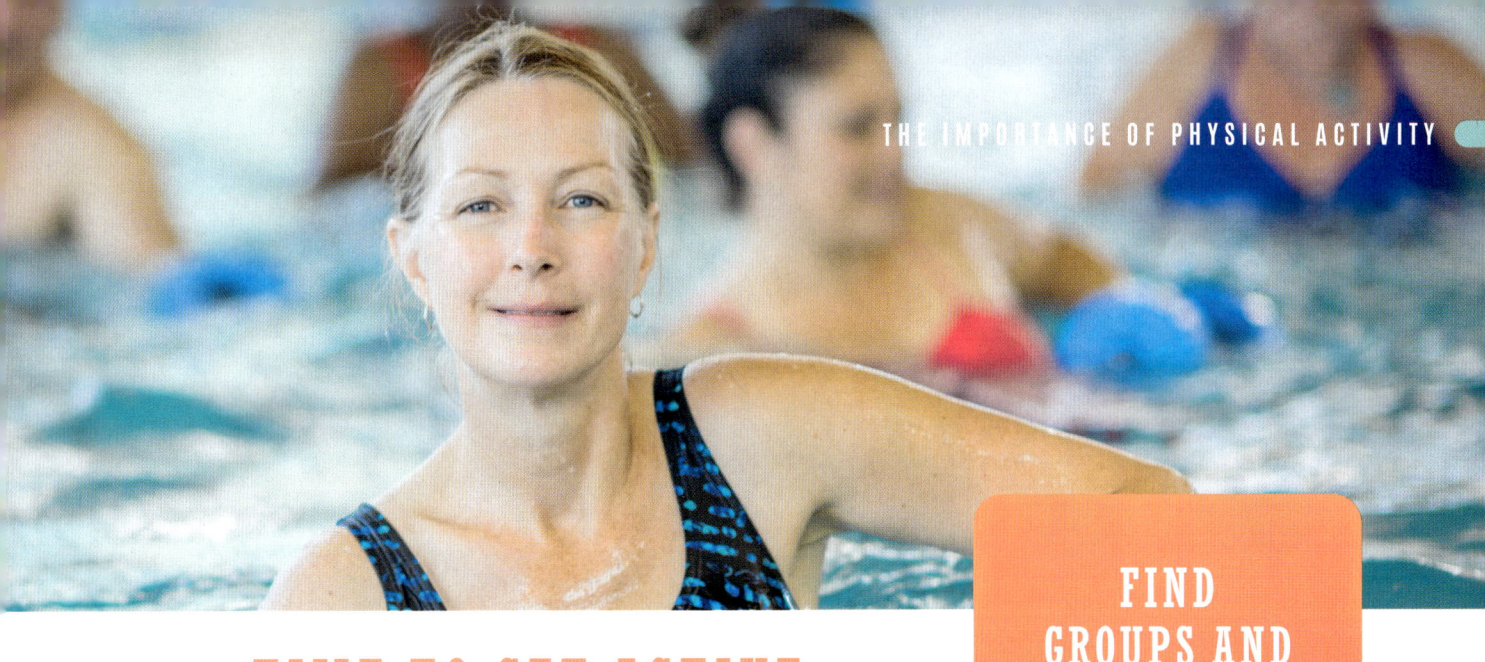

TIME TO GET ACTIVE

Hopefully we've convinced you of the 'why' when it comes to being more active, so now it's time to focus on the 'how'. In the next feature, we'll look at the four best types of exercise for people with high blood pressure, but here are some tips to help you get started!

Start slowly

It's so easy to get caught up in the enthusiasm of a new fitness routine, but if you do too much too soon, you'll end up getting injured or unwell, setting you back to square one. You should only increase your activity by a little bit at a time, and progress from there. Listen to your body, and don't be afraid to step back if you need to, before building up again.

Little and often

Don't be a weekend warrior! It's much better to do a little physical activity every day than to sit down all week and spend a few hours at the weekend working out hard. The prolonged periods of being sedentary are as bad for us as the lack of exercise. By all means, enjoy being active at the weekends, but don't neglect the everyday movement either.

Get some support

Ask your friends and family to help you stay on track. Whether that's by joining you on a walk or just reminding you to get up and move around. Any lifestyle change is made easier when you have people to support you and enable you to meet your goals.

Do what you can

You might be surrounded by expensive gyms, complicated classes and the latest fancy workout gear, but you don't need any of this to succeed. You can be physically active wearing clothes you already own and without spending a penny. Grab your most comfortable shoes and go for a walk around the block, or pop a workout video on YouTube and do it in your pyjamas. Sometimes we get so caught up in doing things the 'right' way, that we end up not doing anything at all. Something is always better than nothing.

FIND GROUPS AND RESOURCES

If you need some help to get started, then there are plenty of ways to get extra support

You don't have to start your fitness journey alone; you might need a little extra help to get going. There are some great apps that you can use to help build your strength and physical fitness. If you want to start running, then why not try a Couch to 5K plan? There are plenty available and they all follow similar principles. You build up very slowly over about nine weeks to be able to run for 30 minutes continuously or a total of five kilometres, depending on the plan. They usually start with about 60 seconds of running with lots of walking in-between and are aimed at beginners. You could also find videos to follow at home on YouTube, use apps to track your walking, or engage the services of a personal trainer at your local gym to help you out. Look for local walking groups and rambling groups too, as these can help you meet new people and keep you motivated.

LIFESTYLE

THE BEST TYPES OF EXERCISE FOR HYPERTENSION

If you're looking to control your blood pressure, these are the top activities to include

MODERATE-INTENSITY CONTINUOUS TRAINING (MICT)

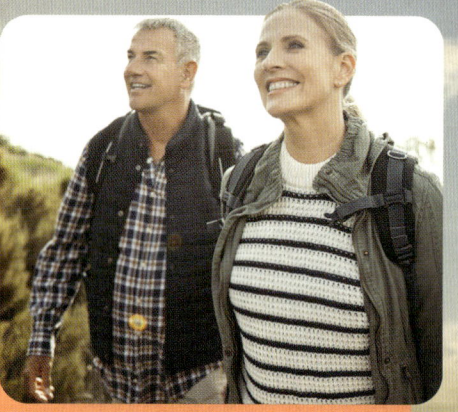

We often hear about HIIT – high-intensity interval training – where you work hard for short periods of time with longer recoveries in between. However, you might hear less about MICT, or moderate-intensity continuous training. This involves doing a longer period of continuous activity at a pace that is considered 'moderate'. This means that you shouldn't feel like you could keep going forever (low intensity) and it shouldn't feel like your heart is racing and you're struggling to draw a breath (high intensity). A moderate intensity should raise your heart rate and respiration rate, but you should still be able to talk. The NHS UK describes it as being the point at which you can still talk, but not sing. MICT is also called aerobic exercise.

When it comes to doing MICT, you want to choose something you enjoy. This could be walking, swimming or cycling, for example. Everyone's fitness is different, so some people may find that they can jog at a pace that keeps them at a moderate intensity, but for others, walking at a good pace is perfectly adequate. As you get fitter, you might have to walk a bit faster or add in some hills to maintain a moderate intensity. That's what's so great about MICT – it works for everyone and is scalable to suit your improving fitness.

Ideally, you want to build up to doing around 30 to 60 minutes of MICT five to seven days a week. That might seem a lot, but you can start off by doing ten minutes a day and go from there. You can also break it up into a few sessions a day, for example, ten minutes of walking three times a day. You could, for example, get into a routine where you walk for ten minutes after each mealtime. This kind of exercise helps to lower your risk of heart disease and reduces your blood pressure.

THE BEST TYPES OF EXERCISE FOR HYPERTENSION

ISOMETRIC EXERCISES

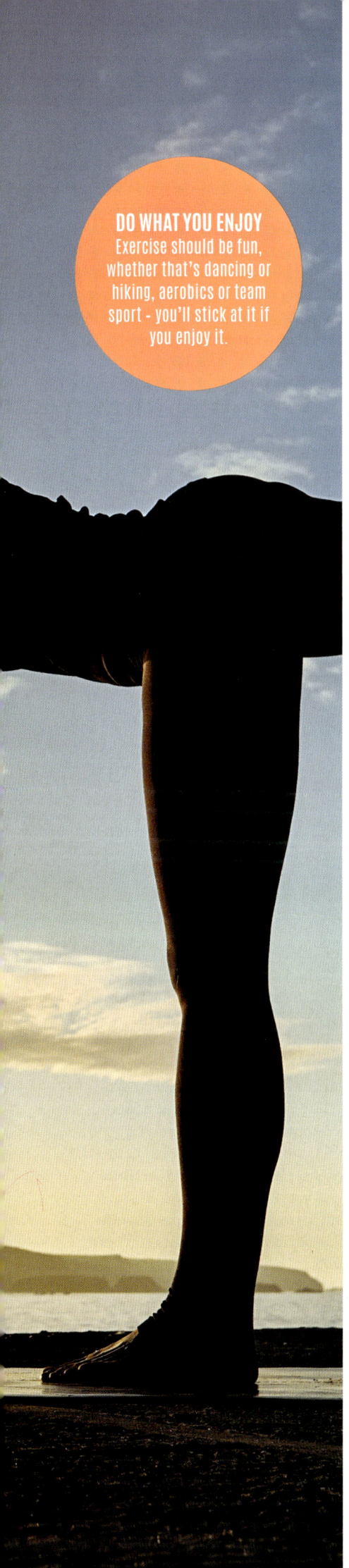

DO WHAT YOU ENJOY
Exercise should be fun, whether that's dancing or hiking, aerobics or team sport - you'll stick at it if you enjoy it.

You might have never heard of the term 'isometric exercise', but you've probably seen examples of them. An isometric exercise is one that keeps a muscle or group of muscles contracted in a static position. This includes things like a plank, a wall squat or a glute bridge. The advantage of these kinds of exercises is that they are low impact and help you build strength. That's not to say they're easy though! There are various modifications and levels of each kind of move – for example, you could do a plank on your knees or come into a shallower squat against a wall.

Isometric exercises can be more suitable for some people than their counterpart, isotonic exercises. Isotonic exercises are also moves that you'll be familiar with, as these involve contracting your muscles and then lengthening them again with movement. This includes things like bicep curls or squats. Isotonic exercises are better overall for building strength, but isometric ones are great for maintaining the muscle strength, for coming back from injury or surgery, and for those newer to strength training.

They are also great for people with hypertension. A 2023 piece of research, published in the British Journal of Sports Medicine, found that these isometric moves were better than other forms of exercise when it comes to lowering blood pressure. One theory is that holding the muscle in a contracted position increases blood flow to the muscles, impacting positively on blood pressure. It came out top of all the exercise types in the research, which included aerobic exercise, resistance training, combined training and high-intensity interval training. However, every single one of these did have a positive impact on blood pressure, so it's good to have a varied and mixed routine. If you're not already, adding in isometric moves is worth doing. You can do them anywhere, anytime, so they're easy to fit into your day – you could even watch TV from a wall squat!

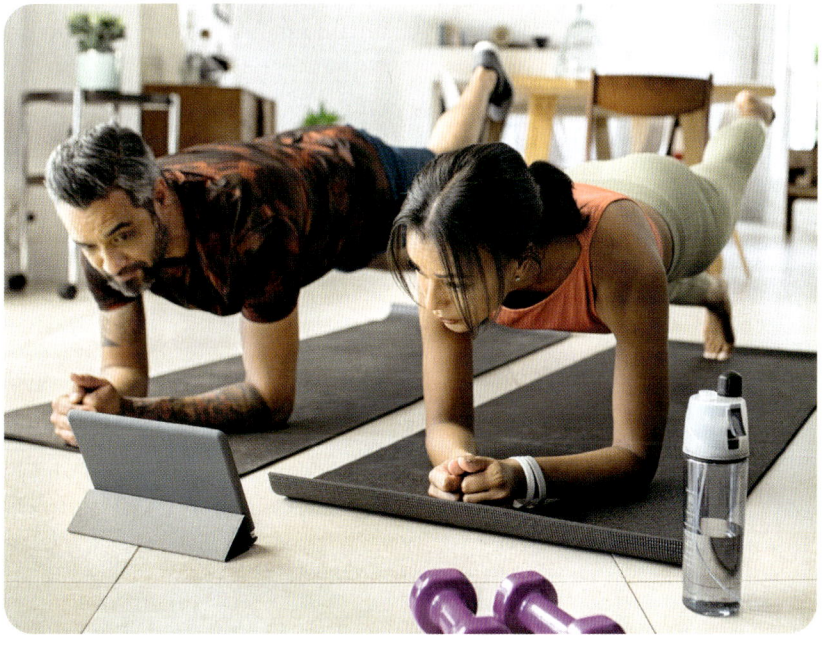

Images Getty

89

LIFESTYLE

RESISTANCE TRAINING

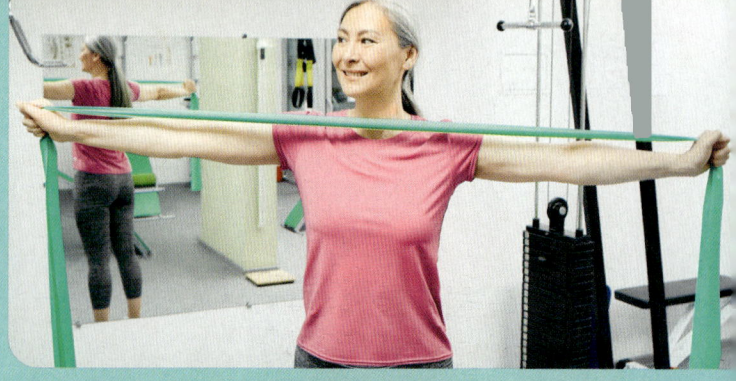

Resistance training is any form of exercise in which you work your muscles against some kind of resistance, otherwise known as strength training.

It's recommended that you aim to do two strength sessions a week, which can help you to build your muscles as well as reduce your blood pressure. It's best to do resistance training, as well as cardiovascular exercise, each week.

Many people feel a bit intimidated when it comes to resistance training and are unsure where to start. But you don't need to be in the gym mastering the weights section from day one. You can start with using just bodyweight to create the resistance you need. Bodyweight exercises can be very effective, and you can begin at a level that works for you. Try including things like lunges, squats, push-ups and tricep dips. You can find free video routines on YouTube to get started, or you could ask a personal trainer to show you some moves.

You may want to progress to using resistance bands, which are cheap, portable and easy to use. These bands come in different strengths so that you can build up, and you can use them to do everything from bicep curls to chest presses. Using resistance bands can also support your muscles and help you become more flexible. They're also good to use from a chair if you have restricted mobility. You could then move on to using dumbbells or kettlebells as you get stronger. If you have access to a gym, you will find a selection of free weights for you to use, as well as assisted weight machines. These machines are great for working the whole body and usually have clear instructions on them to help you get the most out of them.

YOGA

Alongside cardiovascular and strength exercises, the final piece of the fitness puzzle is to do some form of activity that helps you with your flexibility and balance. Yoga is perfect for this, as it is accessible for most people and there are lots of different types of yoga to suit everyone. Start with a beginner class if you've never done it before so that you can get used to the moves and ensure you're doing it properly. If you have high blood pressure, you can take breaks between poses if you need to, and try to move slowly from one position to another.

A key part of yoga is the breathing. It can be instinctual to hold your breath when you're in a pose, but this will raise your blood pressure even more than the move itself. When you're in a pose, you should breathe deeply to help your muscles relax. You may need to be more careful with poses that involve inversion, where your head is lower than your heart, as this can make you feel lightheaded or dizzy. There are plenty of poses that will help you to build strength and flexibility, as well as improve your balance, without inversion.

There are quite a few studies that show a link between yoga and lower blood pressure. One article, published in BMC Public Health in 2022, explored the 'antihypertensive effects of yoga in general patient population' and wrote: 'The odds of having normal blood pressure and using yoga were 85% greater than the odds of having normal blood pressure and not using yoga'. Yoga can help to reduce stress, improve sleep and boost your energy – all of which will also have a positive impact on blood pressure.

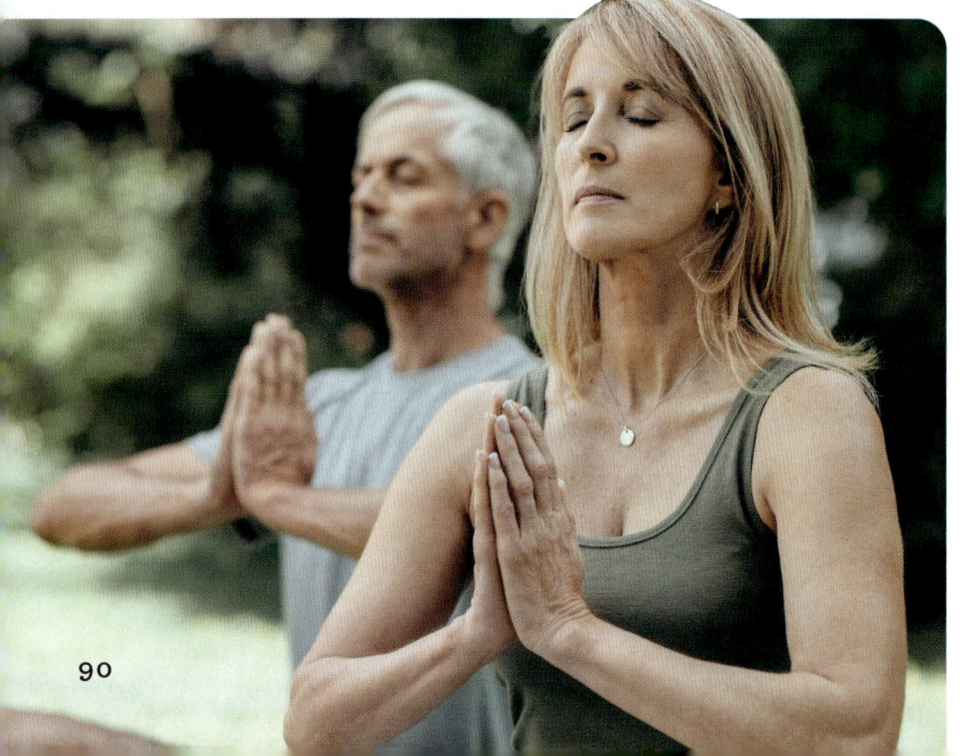

THE BEST TYPES OF EXERCISE FOR HYPERTENSION

WHAT ABOUT WEIGHTLIFTING?

Advice on lifting heavy weights is mixed, but if in doubt, ask your doctor

Most sources agree that resistance training and weight training are great and beneficial forms of exercise for people with high blood pressure. However, when it comes to lifting heavy, the response is more mixed. It depends on how high your blood pressure is and whether it's well controlled, as well as your overall fitness level and ability. When you lift something especially heavy, it can lead to a sudden and intense spike in your blood pressure, something that can be more dangerous for someone with uncontrolled, severe hypertension. It's better to start off with smaller weights and higher repetitions, building weight slowly as you get used to the exercise. As your blood pressure improves, you can look at increasing your weights more. You may benefit from working with a personal trainer to ensure that your technique is correct and that you're breathing properly (many people hold their breath when lifting something heavy) before lifting bigger weights to get the best out of each move, as well as look after your health.

SET A CHALLENGE

Entering an event or setting a challenge can help you to stay motivated long term

Having a goal can help you stay on track with your exercise and give you something to work towards. For example, you may want to enter an event, such as a running, walking, cycling or swimming event. This could be a long-distance walk, a Parkrun (a weekly, free, timed 5K run held in local parks), a race or other fitness challenge. Having an event gives you a clear timeline of when you need to meet your goal, as well as encouraging you to push yourself. You can put in place a training plan that builds you up from where you are now to where you need to be, so you can see your progress as you go through it week by week. You might prefer a challenge where you can tick off what you've achieved every day – a month-long challenge is perfect to commit to. You might aim to walk 10,000 steps a day for 30 days, for example, or do 20 minutes of some kind of activity a day.

KNOW WHEN TO STOP
If you feel ill, dizzy or faint, or have any pain, then pause your workout and seek medical advice.

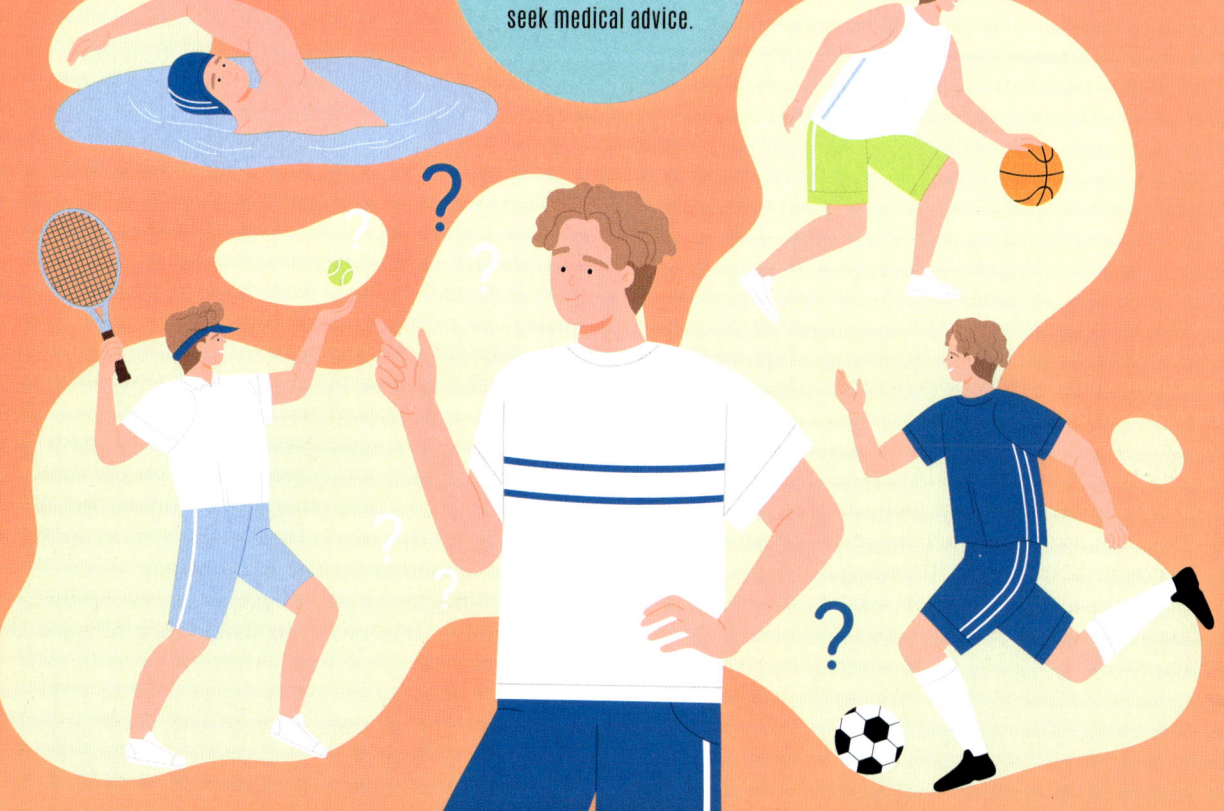

91

LIFESTYLE

IMPROVE YOUR SLEEP

Getting enough good-quality sleep can help you when you're aiming to reduce your blood pressure

We need sleep. It's absolutely essential to our body to keep everything functioning as it should. Getting the right amount of sleep, and good-quality sleep, helps to protect our physical, emotional and mental health. When you're making lifestyle changes to help with your blood pressure, paying attention to your sleep should be part of your treatment plan.

Can sleep impact on blood pressure?

Most adults need somewhere between seven and nine hours of sleep a night. We're all different, so some of us will fall at the lower end of that range and some higher. It's not unusual to have the odd bad night of sleep – you might be worried about something, have a late night out, be away from home, be under a lot of stress, or have jet lag, for example. A night, or even a few nights, of bad sleep will make you feel a bit grumpy, less focused and low in energy the next day and for a couple of days after. However, a short-term sleep disruption won't affect your long-term health, and getting back to good sleep again as soon as possible will be enough to undo the side effects.

The problems begin when you have more bad nights than good. Long-term issues with sleep have been linked to poorer health. In particular, if you get less than five to six hours' sleep regularly, you are more likely to become overweight or obese, develop diabetes or get heart disease. People with poor sleep – whether that's not enough sleep, interrupted sleep or insomnia – are also more likely to have high blood pressure. Some research shows that this link to hypertension is worse in middle age and in women. One study[1] tracked the health of more than 65,000 women, all aged between 25 to 42 and without hypertension at the start, for 16 years. It found that women who slept for five or six hours a night were between 7-10% more likely to develop hypertension in comparison to those who slept for seven to eight hours. And women with insomnia were between 14-28% more likely to have hypertension than those who rarely had trouble sleeping.

We don't know that sleep itself is a direct cause of hypertension, but some of the risk factors for high blood pressure can also lead to problems with sleep. For example, those who are overweight or obese are more likely to have sleep apnoea. People who are under a lot of stress might struggle to sleep too, and the stress could contribute to elevated blood pressure. Plus, when you're not sleeping, you might not feel like exercising as much or making healthy food choices.

When you sleep, your blood pressure should naturally drop,

PRIORITISE SLEEP
Be strict with your sleep schedule – it's so important for your overall health and wellbeing.

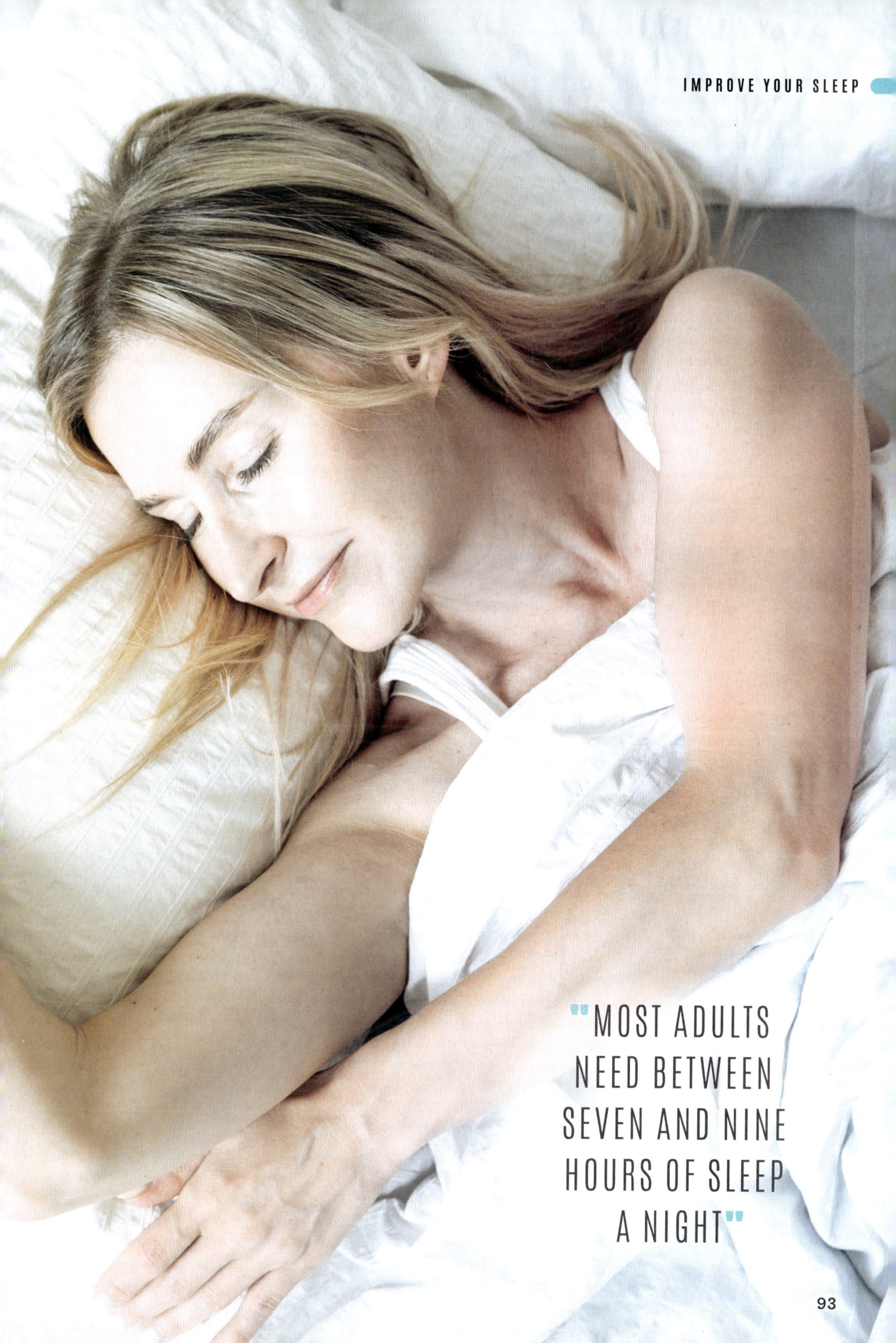

IMPROVE YOUR SLEEP

"MOST ADULTS NEED BETWEEN SEVEN AND NINE HOURS OF SLEEP A NIGHT"

LIFESTYLE

called 'nocturnal dipping'. This can be anything from 10-20% lower than your normal daytime readings. Health problems can occur in people whose blood pressure dips more than 20% or less than 10%. If your blood pressure doesn't drop as much as it should at night, you might be at a higher risk of heart disease and stroke.

It can be difficult for those who work a shift pattern that involves nights, as this can be very disruptive to sleep. While there is no concrete evidence about a specific link between hypertension and shift work, there are research studies linking shift patterns to other health problems like being overweight, having high cholesterol and developing diabetes – which can, in turn, impact blood pressure.

Why sleep matters

Sleep deprivation impacts us in lots of different ways. You might find that you are less alert, have slower reaction times or find it hard to concentrate. This can make it difficult to do everyday things, such as driving or working. You might also have lower mood, anxiety or depression; do less socialising; and feel irritable.

When we're asleep, there is a lot going on in our brains and bodies. For example, your body uses the downtime to repair and rebuild itself, helping you to heal from injury and illness, as well as doing general maintenance. This includes giving the brain time to process the day and sort your memories into short and long term. It also gives your heart a chance to rest and repair any damage. Getting enough sleep can reduce inflammation in the body too, and help prevent fatty deposits from building up in the arteries that lead to the heart. Sleep also helps to regulate your hormones and blood sugar levels, and is important to your immune system function. You're more likely to pick up viruses and infections when you're run down from a lack of sleep.

Another benefit of sleep is that it helps with your mental health and improves your mood. It can help with focus and attention, as well as your energy levels. When you've had enough sleep, you wake up feeling more ready to face the day. A lack of sleep is linked to being overweight and not eating properly. When you're awake for longer your body needs more energy – ie food – which can lead to overeating, and when you're tired, you might not want to spend time preparing and cooking a full meal.

With good sleep, we're more likely to make good decisions and stay motivated. This is especially important as you embark on a healthy lifestyle to help reduce your blood pressure – getting good sleep is going to help you meet all your other goals.

How to get better sleep

So, we know that sleep is important, but what do you do if you're struggling to get enough? First, you need to address any underlying issues that might be preventing you from getting a good night's sleep. That could be because of a sleep disorder (see the box on the next page), a partner snoring, or too much light coming in to your room. It's not always easy to solve these kinds of problems, but you can try things like speaking to a doctor for medication to help with sleep disorders, wearing earplugs or investing in a good eye mask. Some reasons that we're not getting enough sleep are unavoidable, such as working at night or having a small baby. You can only do the best you can in the time you have available to sleep, and you need to optimise your hours in bed.

Having a good sleep routine can help to prepare your body for rest. Some people like to read before bed or have a warm shower. Ideally, put your phone away at least an hour before bed and do something else. Turn the lights down low to signal to your body that it's almost time to go to bed. Try to go to bed and wake up at roughly the same time every day so that you fall into a rhythm. Ideally, you don't want to eat too close to bedtime, or drink alcohol, both of which can prevent you from sleeping. You also want to exercise far enough away from your usual rest time, to give your body time to calm down. Make sure that you have a dark, cool environment to sleep in, and that you're comfortable.

Your lifestyle choices can also aid sleep. If you are physically active, get plenty of fresh air, drink lots of water and eat a healthy diet, this can all help you to sleep properly. These also all help with lowering blood pressure, so you can see how lifestyle interventions really do work from every angle.

> "HAVING A GOOD SLEEP ROUTINE CAN HELP PREPARE YOUR BODY FOR REST"

SLEEP DISORDERS

Some people find it harder to sleep than others, which may be due to an underlying sleep disorder

There may be a reason why you're not getting enough sleep. Some people have sleep disorders that prevent them from getting a healthy and balanced amount of good-quality sleep. This includes sleep apnoea, which we've already discussed in our section on secondary hypertension. We know that people who have this sleeping disorder, which causes difficulty breathing at night, are more likely to develop hypertension. It's most likely in people who are very overweight, and it's more common in men than women.

Another sleep disorder is insomnia, which is when you regularly have trouble with getting to sleep or staying asleep. Many people will suffer from insomnia, and it usually passes, but those with chronic insomnia have trouble with sleep at least three times a week for at least three months. There are some studies that suggest a link between insomnia and a heightened risk of hypertension.

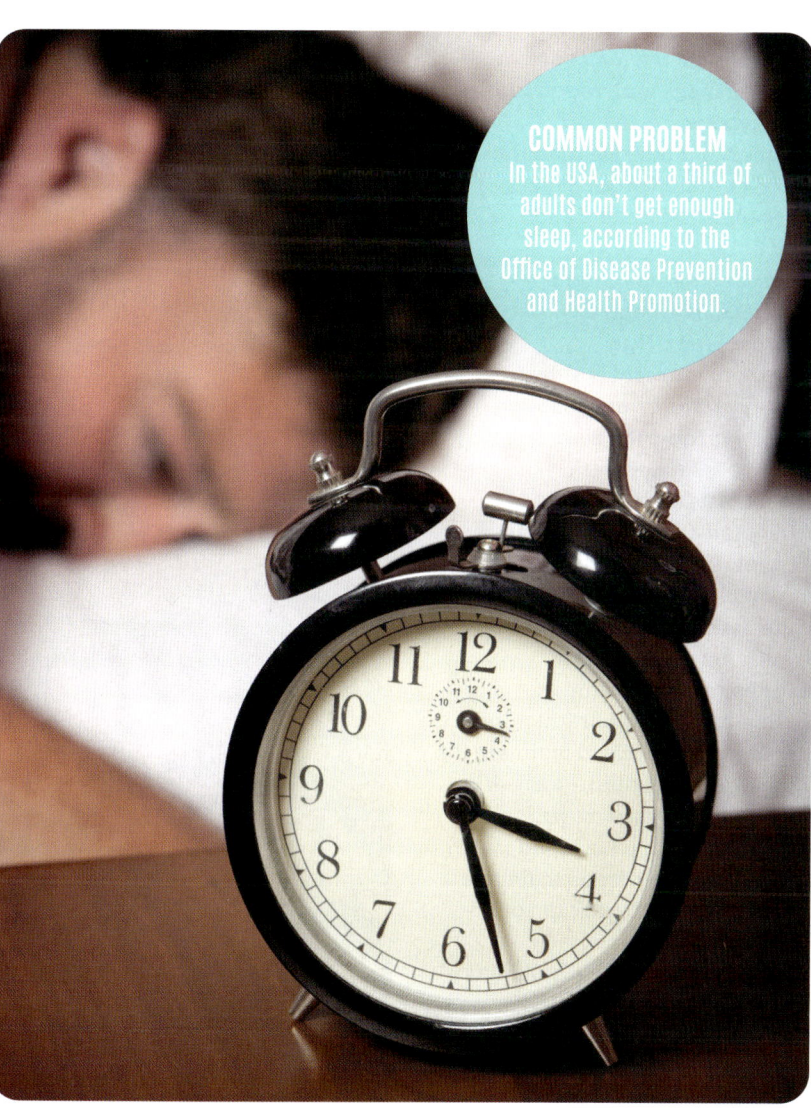

COMMON PROBLEM
In the USA, about a third of adults don't get enough sleep, according to the Office of Disease Prevention and Health Promotion.

IMPROVE YOUR SLEEP

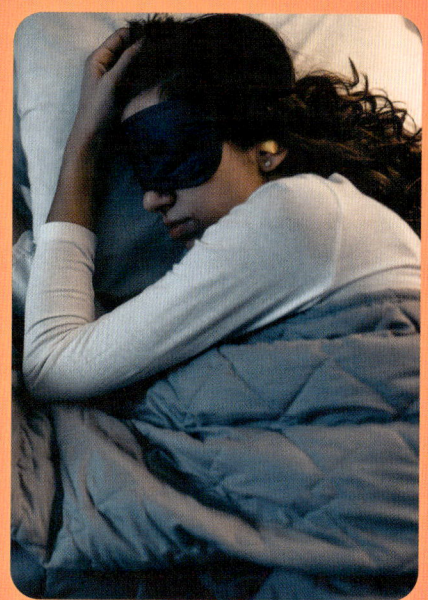

TOO MUCH SLEEP

Getting the right amount of sleep means not getting too much or too little

It can be tempting to try to claw back lost sleep by spending longer in bed or adding in naps, but there is some evidence that shows too much sleep has as much impact on our health as too little sleep does. Oversleeping can lead to symptoms like drowsiness, fatigue and anxiety in the short term. As with not getting enough sleep, the odd night of oversleeping won't do you any harm, but chronic oversleeping has been linked to poorer mental health and a higher risk of some health conditions. Too much sleep can also be linked to weight gain and higher blood sugar levels. One research paper[2] looked at numerous studies exploring the link between sleep and hypertension and concluded that: 'Excessively longer and shorter periods of sleep may both be risk factors for high blood pressure; these associations are stronger in women than men'.

[1] *Hypertension* journal, November 2023. [2] Relationship between Duration of Sleep and Hypertension in Adults: A Meta-Analysis. Journal of Clinical Sleep Medicine, September 2015.

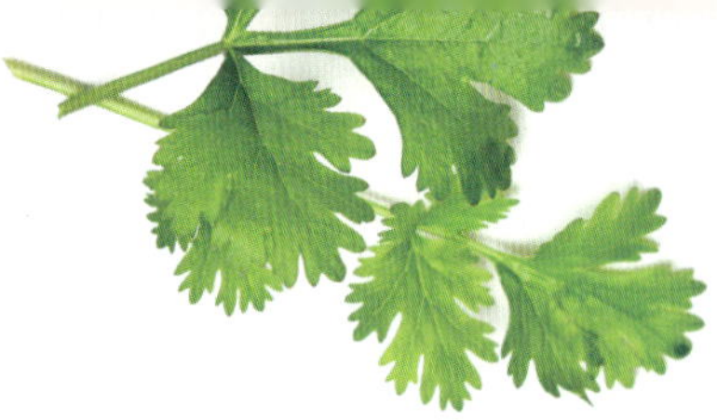

LIFESTYLE

HOW TO EAT FOR HYPERTENSION

What you eat can have a massive impact on blood pressure. We explain what you should be including and reducing in your diet

When you've been diagnosed with hypertension, you may be looking at changing or optimising your diet to help support your body and lower your blood pressure. Generally speaking, eating a healthy and balanced diet, full of whole foods and low in processed foods, will give your body the support it needs. However, many of us need more guidance on how to build a healthy and balanced diet, and what foods need to be reduced or avoided completely.

If you prefer to follow a food style or plan, to give you inspiration and education around what you should be eating, you could look at either the Mediterranean diet or the DASH diet. The Mediterranean diet is often called the 'best diet in the world', thanks to its balanced approach, backed up by numerous studies about its contribution to better health outcomes. It has been shown to help lower blood pressure, protect the heart and reduce cholesterol levels. It puts the focus on eating plenty of fruits and vegetables, wholegrains, beans and legumes, a moderate amount of low-fat dairy products, fish, poultry and nuts, and very limited sugary, processed or fatty foods.

The DASH (Dietary Approaches to Stop Hypertension) diet is similar in its approach, but it also directly targets the risk factors associated with hypertension. The basic principles are the same as the Mediterranean diet, but it also emphasises lowering salt intake, while eating foods that are high in potassium, calcium and magnesium. Potassium in particular is an important mineral, as it helps the body to maintain the right balance of fluid – excess fluid puts pressure on your blood vessels, raising your blood pressure. Eating foods that have a lot of potassium can help your kidneys to work optimally, especially important if salt intake is high. It's better to get potassium from food rather than supplements, as you can have too much potassium, which can then

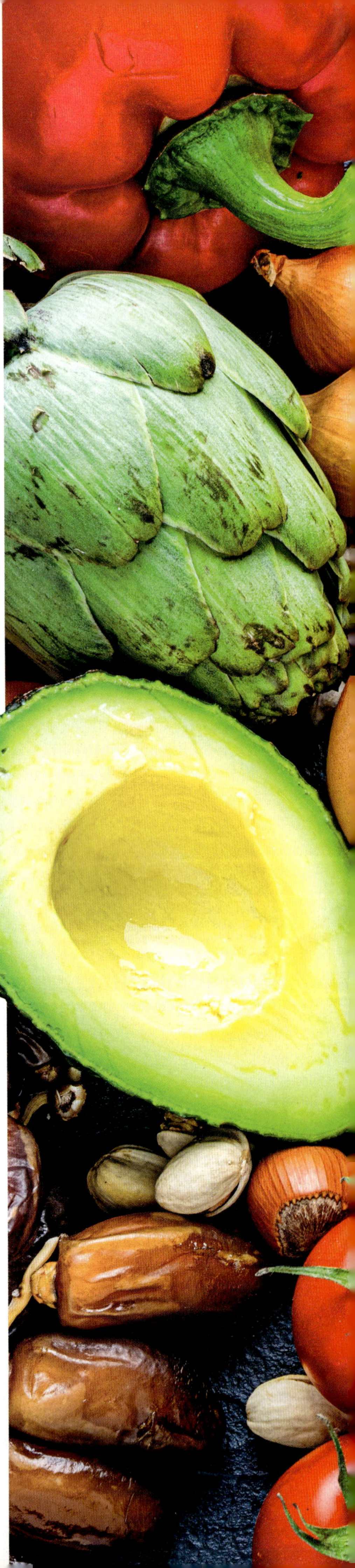

> "THE MEDITERRANEAN DIET IS OFTEN CALLED THE 'BEST DIET IN THE WORLD'"

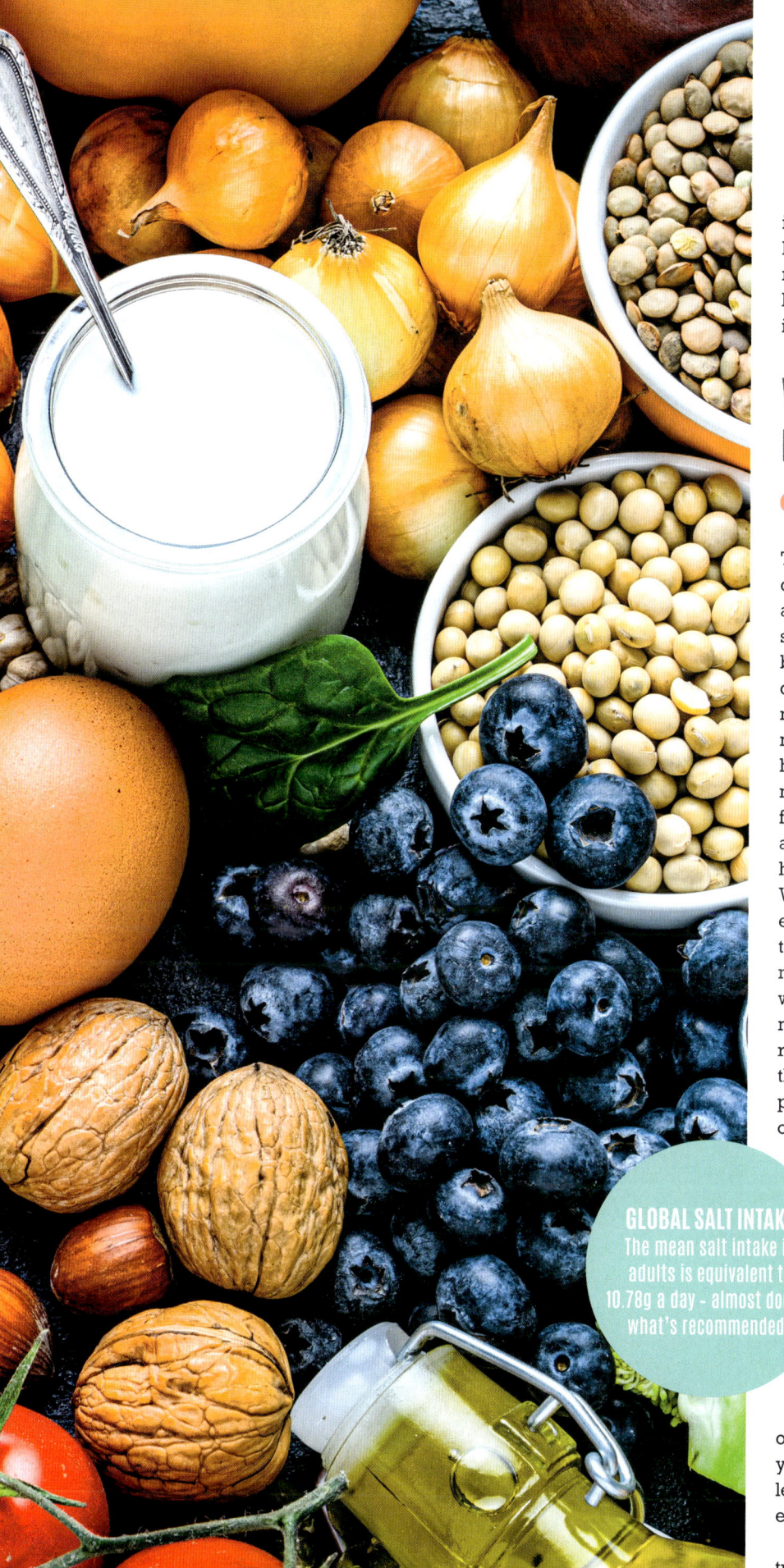

HOW TO EAT FOR HYPERTENSION

impact on your kidneys. If you have kidney disease, you may need to speak to your doctor before increasing your potassium intake too heavily.

What you need to know about salt

The most important thing that you can do in your diet is to reduce the amount of salt you eat. We know that salt increases blood pressure and by cutting it from your diet, you could begin to see results within months. If you take blood pressure medicine, but continue to eat a diet high in salt, then the treatment may not work as effectively, therefore following a low-salt approach is advised for everyone with high blood pressure. When we eat salt, it encourages the body to hold on to fluid. We need a little salt, but when we eat too much, our body retains more fluid than it should, and this puts pressure on the blood vessels.

You might think that you don't eat much salt if you're not actively adding salt to your meals or during cooking, but unfortunately salt is hidden in so many common foods that you could be consuming far more than you should without realising. And all types of salt are the same in terms of your intake, so it doesn't matter if you're using processed table salt or less processed rock salt, for example. It all adds up.

It can be helpful to use a food-tracking app for a few weeks and logging everything you eat. You can then see what your daily average intake of salt is right now. The recommendation for healthy

GLOBAL SALT INTAKE
The mean salt intake in adults is equivalent to 10.78g a day – almost double what's recommended.[1]

[1] World Health Organization. **Images** Getty

LIFESTYLE

salt intake is no more than 6g, which is about a level teaspoon. Where it gets confusing is that sometimes you will see a guide for salt and sometimes a guide for sodium. Salt is sodium chloride, and it is the sodium value that contributes to blood pressure problems. That means that if you see a weight for salt, that will include both the sodium and the chloride. 6g of salt is the same as about 2.4g of sodium, which is usually expressed as 2400mg. When you're checking nutritional food labels, you need to know whether you're looking at a sodium value or a salt value. If you have very high blood pressure, you may be given a different salt or sodium target to help get it under control.

When you're cooking at home with fresh ingredients, you have a little more control over your salt intake. Try to avoid adding salt during the cooking process. You can add flavour with other herbs and spices instead. Be careful if you're using things like stock cubes, pre-made sauces or gravies, as these are often heavy in salt. However, around 75% of the salt we eat every day is hidden in the foods that we buy, including soy sauce, pickles, table sauces, cheese, bacon, bread, processed meats, cereals, ready-made sandwiches, ready meals, sausages and ready-made soups. You will need to get used to reading product labels to see how much salt is inside, and choosing lower-salt alternatives. Usually you will see a 'per 100g' value, which helps you to compare one product with another. There should also be a value for one serving, so that you can work out how much you're eating. You should try to prepare your own food at home as much as possible.

> "TRY TO AVOID ADDING SALT DURING THE COOKING PROCESS"

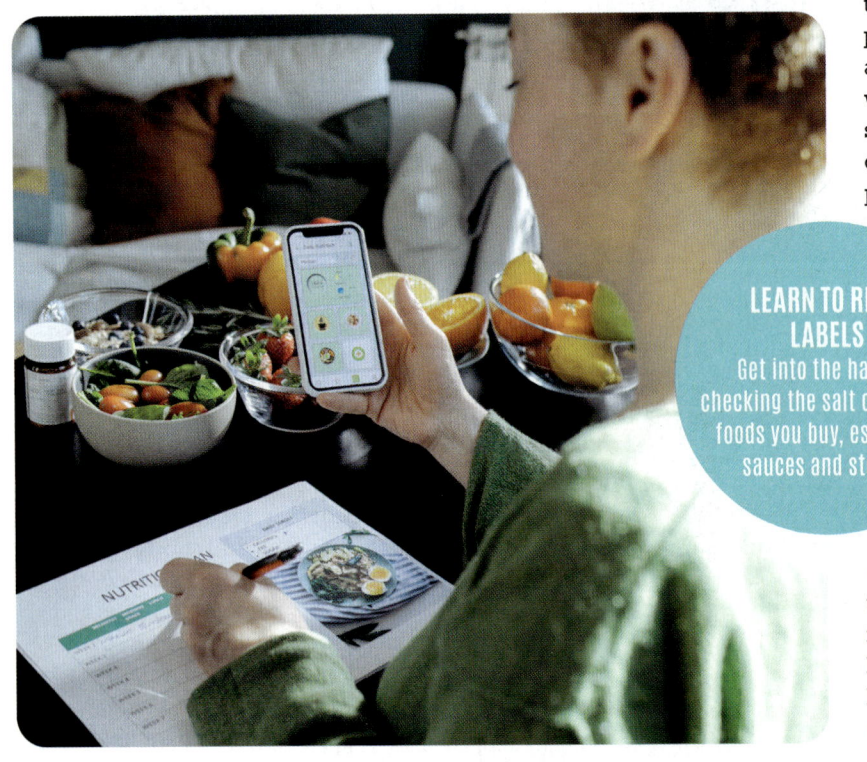

LEARN TO READ LABELS
Get into the habit of checking the salt content of foods you buy, especially sauces and stocks.

Fruits and vegetables

You should be looking at increasing the amount of fruit and vegetables you eat. The 'five a day' figure is a great target, but this is considered the minimum. Try to make sure that you're eating a wide variety of products, as they each have different properties and nutrients, helping to support your overall health. Vegetables are great for filling your plate at mealtimes, so try to get a couple of different varieties in per meal, whether that's adding a big salad or cooking two to three different vegetables to go with your protein and carbohydrates. Fruit makes a great topping for porridge and is the perfect, portable snack. A portion of fruit is considered to be about 80g, but you don't have to weigh everything. For medium-sized fruits (like an apple or orange), then one piece of fruit is a portion; for smaller fruits (like plums or apricots), you need two pieces per portion. A portion is also three heaped tablespoons of vegetables, berries or pulses; a small bowl of salad; or a tablespoon of dried fruit.

We've already mentioned how important it is to get potassium in your diet, and this can be achieved through your fruit and vegetable intake. Try to include some high-potassium foods every day. For fruits, this includes apricots (fresh or dried), raisins, dates,

HOW TO EAT FOR HYPERTENSION

WHAT ABOUT DRINKS?

Don't forget to consider what you're drinking when you're looking at adapting your diet

We can often forget to think about our drinks as part of overall dietary changes. The best thing to drink is water, as this helps our body to work properly and flush our systems. Ideally, we should all be drinking at least six to eight glasses of water per day. When you're dehydrated, your body will hold on to more sodium, which can then cause high blood pressure. If you find it hard to drink enough plain water, you could add in a slice of lemon or lime for extra flavour. You could also have sparkling water if you prefer.

It's perfectly fine to have some tea or coffee, but be careful what you're adding things to them. It's best to have hot drinks without sugar where possible, and you may wish to switch to lower-fat milk. Caffeine can have a short-term impact on blood pressure, so limit these drinks to no more than three to four cups per day. When you're watching your sugar and fat intake, don't forget to include soft drinks and alcohol into your daily tracking, as these can often be high in both.

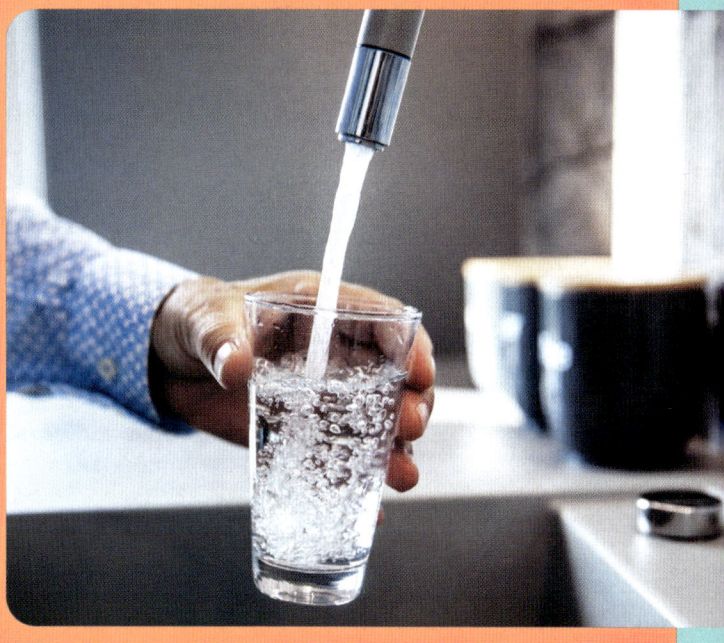

LEARN TO READ A NUTRITIONAL LABEL

Food labels can be confusing, but you'll need to get to grips with them

All packaged foods should carry a nutritional label on them by law. This will give you a breakdown of the important nutrients and how much there is of each. These will often have both a 'per 100g' figure, as well as a 'per serving' figure. However, sometimes you will need to work out the amount per serving yourself. Pay attention to what the serving is, as it might be smaller than you think. The key values to look at include the number of calories in the product (particularly if you're trying to lose weight); this is usually expressed first as an energy value in kilojoules (kj) and then as a calorie value (kcal), so make sure you read the right one! Next, look at how much fat is in the product – there should be a separate saturated fat value – and the sugar value, which comes under carbohydrates. Finally, the other key metric is the amount of salt, which is expressed in g or mg. Some foods may have a traffic-light label on them, which gives a visual guide as to whether a food is healthier (green), moderately healthy (amber) or less healthy (red).

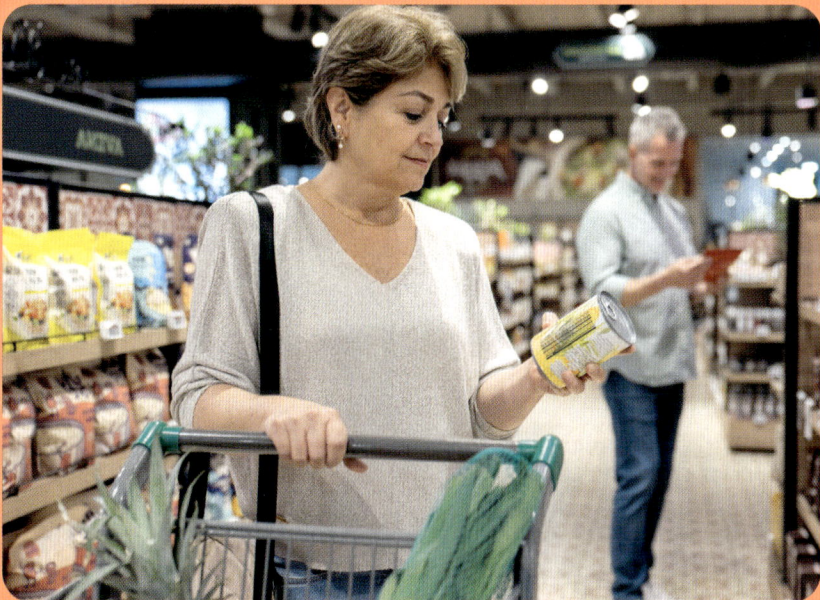

LIFESTYLE

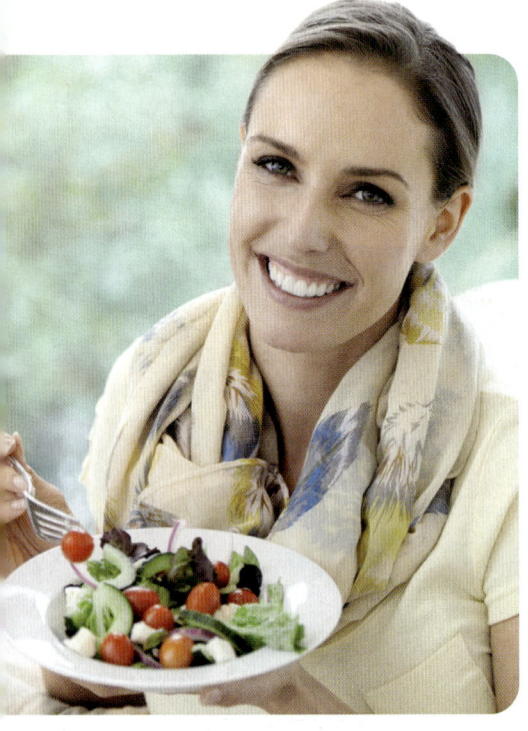

"IF YOU EAT MEAT, THEN TRY TO CHOOSE LEANER CUTS TO CUT DOWN ON SATURATED FAT"

Wholegrains and protein

Both wholegrains and protein are important in your diet. Wholegrains are grains that include the whole of the grain kernel, as opposed to simple grains that are stripped. The advantage of wholegrains is that they can help to increase potassium in the body, which we know lowers blood pressure, as well as protect the blood vessels. They are also packed with other essential nutrients, supporting whole-body health, and they can help with decreasing the risk of insulin resistance. They are also good for your fibre intake. Fibre helps you to feel fuller for longer, which is good if you're also trying to lose weight. Eating enough fibre is shown to help reduce the risk of heart disease, stroke, diabetes and some cancers. As an adult, the recommended amount of fibre is around 30g per day, but many of us eat less than this.

Wholegrains include things like wholegrain versions of pasta, bread and cereal, as well as barley, rye bread, millet, oats, wild rice and quinoa. You can start by doing some simple swaps, such as white bread for wholegrain bread. Ideally you should have at least three servings of around 30g each per day to boost your health.

It's also important to have protein in your diet, which should come from lean, unprocessed sources where possible. Protein comes from both animal and plant sources. If you eat meat, then try and choose leaner cuts to cut down on saturated fat. Eating too much red meat has been linked to poorer health outcomes too, so try and limit this to one or two days a week. Poultry, fish and eggs are great sources of animal protein. But you should also include

bananas, oranges (or orange juice), tomatoes (or tomato juice/puree), tropical fruits and melons. For vegetables, this includes potatoes, sweet potatoes, carrots, leafy green vegetables and asparagus.

It doesn't have to be fresh fruit and vegetables either. You can have dried, canned or frozen as well. Frozen fruit and vegetables in particular can be good for shopping on a budget – you can buy a big bag and just use what you need. Also, they are usually frozen quickly after picking, meaning that they are full of nutrients. You can have fruit or vegetable juice, but you should limit this to one glass – it's always better to eat the whole fruit. Some root vegetables are starches and don't count towards your 'five a day', such as potatoes, yams and plantain, but many root vegetables do count. That's not to say you shouldn't eat them – as we've mentioned, potatoes are a great source of potassium – but that you need to add more vegetables to your plate as well.

CHECK YOUR MEDICATION
Make sure you find out if there are any foods you can't have when taking certain medicines.

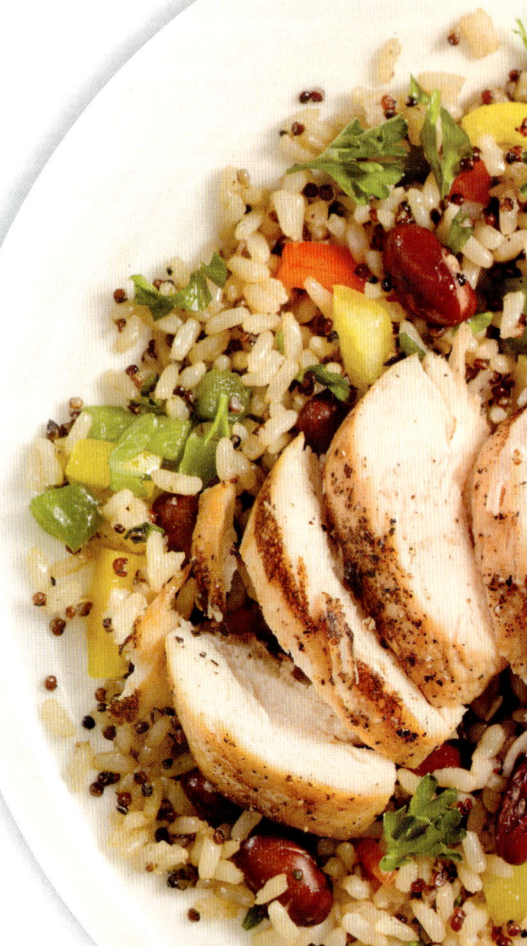

100

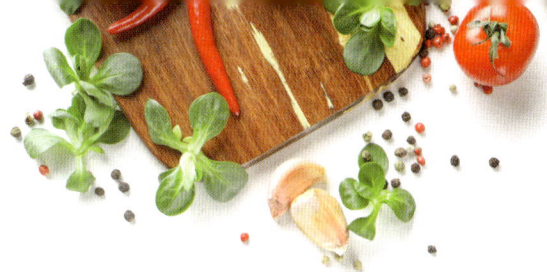

HOW TO EAT FOR HYPERTENSION

some plant protein in your diet, maybe committing to a number of meat-free days. Plant protein sources include legumes and pulses, grains, nuts and seeds, quinoa, tofu, tempeh and soy milk. There is also protein in some fruits and vegetables. It's best to avoid processed 'fake meat' products, as these are often very high in fat and salt.

Fat and sugar

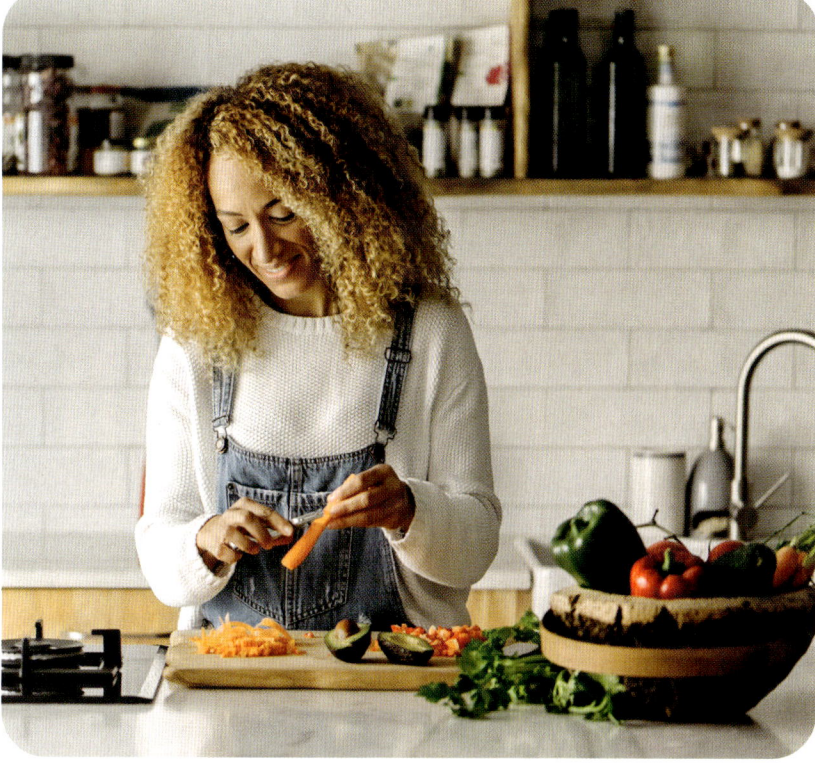

Our bodies do need some fat, as this helps our bodies to work optimally and absorb all the nutrients we need. Unsaturated fats are good for your heart health and can lower your cholesterol, so you do want to be eating some of these. This includes things like olive oil, avocados, nuts and oily fish.

However, it's important to lower your intake of other fats, such as saturated fats and trans fats. These fats can raise your cholesterol levels, narrowing your blood vessels and raising your blood pressure. Saturated fat is found in foods like red meat, processed meat, butter, cheese, cream, pastries, biscuits, crackers and chocolate. Trans fats are found in 'hydrogenated vegetable oils', which may be added to some ultraprocessed products. It's currently recommended to eat no more than 20g (women) or 30g (men) of saturated fat per day.

Eating high-sugar foods can have an impact on your weight, which we know influences your blood pressure, and it can also contribute towards developing type 2 diabetes. We do need some sugar in our bodies for energy, brain function and organ health, however we can get sugar from things like fruit and milk, where it occurs naturally. When we talk about reducing our sugar intake, we're talking about sugar that's added to our food and drink, rather than those naturally occurring sugars.

Ideally, you should be eating less than 30g of sugar per day, which is around seven teaspoons. Unfortunately, processed foods can have much more than this in just one serving. A standard 330ml (or 12oz) can of Coca-Cola, for example, has 35g of sugar. Other food sources of sugar include things like jam, sweets, chocolate, biscuits, cakes and fruit juice, plus of course any sugar you add to tea and coffee. You might also be surprised to find sugar in savoury products, like bread, table sauces and ready meals.

When it comes to eating to reduce your blood pressure, you need to be both adding in the right foods and reducing the wrong ones. It can take time to adjust, especially if your diet is significantly different to this right now. However, every reduction in processed foods and every addition of nutrient-dense foods is a step in the right direction.

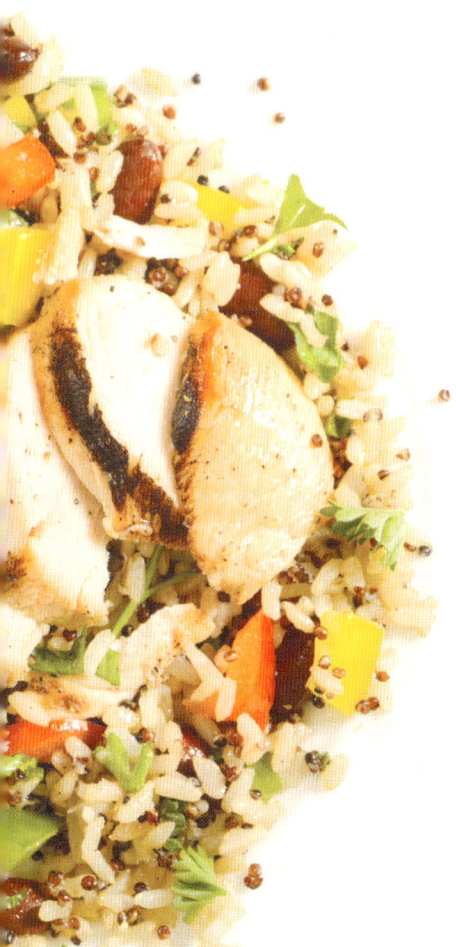
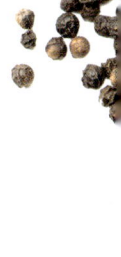

LIFESTYLE

TOP 10 FOODS FOR HYPERTENSION

Include these in your diet to get all the health benefits while helping to reduce your blood pressure

LEAFY GREEN VEGETABLES

Adding leafy green vegetables to your meals is amazing for your overall health. This includes things like cabbage, kale, spinach, rocket and watercress. They are relatively cheap and easy to get hold of throughout the year, and can be added to salads or main meals to bump up your nutrients. These veggie powerhouses are packed with goodness, especially minerals like potassium, magnesium and calcium. We already know that potassium plays a huge role in blood pressure management, but the other minerals are just as important. Magnesium helps blood vessels relax by managing nitric oxide levels, while calcium works on the muscle cells that line the artery walls. Leafy greens also give you plenty of vitamin C, which is an antioxidant; a good amount of fibre; and carotenoids, which are good for heart health. You want to retain as many of the nutrients as possible, so consider steaming or sauteing, rather than boiling, to preserve the goodness. Rocket and watercress, for example, are great to have raw in salads, whereas kale or cabbage are perfect for cooking in a splash of olive oil with added garlic for a taste boost. Try to eat a variety of leafy greens to get a diverse intake of the different minerals and nutrients.

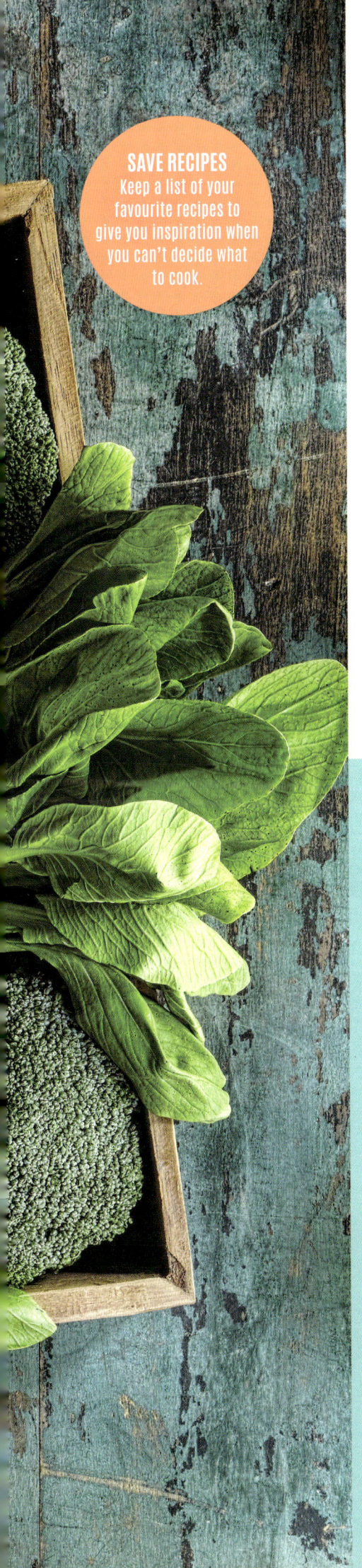

TOP 10 FOODS FOR HYPERTENSION

SAVE RECIPES
Keep a list of your favourite recipes to give you inspiration when you can't decide what to cook.

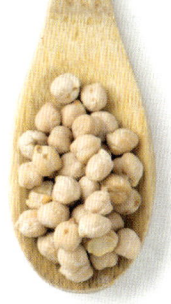
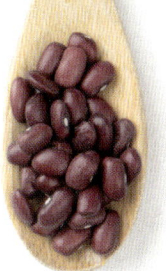

LENTILS AND PULSES

Lentils and pulses are a great addition to a healthy, balanced diet. They are a cheap source of protein and can help to bulk out meals, or even be the star of the show. There are so many different varieties to choose from, and you can buy them fresh, dried or tinned. Tinned beans are ready to use, so they are a quick and simple way to boost your nutrients – think kidney beans, chickpeas and black beans. You can use these to make a tasty three-bean chilli, for example. As well as being high in protein, pulses and lentils are also a good source of fibre and low in fat, making them a great option if you're trying to lose or maintain weight. You do need to check the label to make sure that no salt has been added, and try to choose beans that are stored in water. Sadly, things like baked beans are very salty due to the sauce they are in, but you can learn to make your own version, which is just as tasty but with more health benefits. The same goes for things like hummus – shop-bought options can be packed with salt and fat, but you can make it yourself in minutes with chickpeas and a blender!

BANANAS

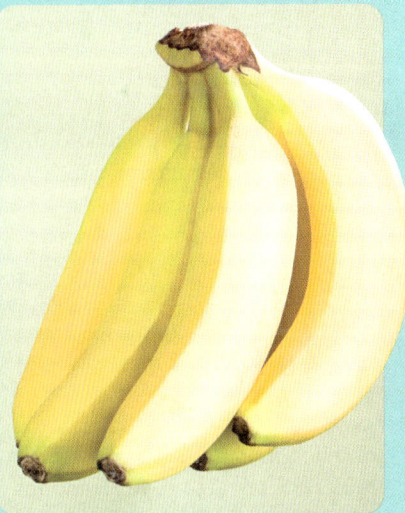

The humble banana is a great fruit to add to your diet when you're managing hypertension. This is because it is packed with potassium, which we know helps with blood pressure by controlling the balance of fluids in the body. A banana contains over 300mg of potassium per 100g (the recommended amount for an adult is about 3,500mg a day) and it's best to get your potassium intake from the foods you eat. As well as being a good source of potassium, bananas are also high in fibre and can help you to feel fuller, so they make a great snack. They're also good for your gut function and energy levels – there's a reason that many people have a banana before or after exercise! They contain a substance called tryptophan, which can help with relaxation and improved mood, so they can make a great pre-bed snack if you feel hungry in the evenings. It's best to have your bananas as they come, but you could also make some healthy banana bread or muffins as a sweet treat. Most people can have bananas without any problems, but if you have kidney disease and have been advised to follow a low-potassium diet, then you may have to limit how many you eat.

LIFESTYLE

DARK CHOCOLATE

If you miss the sweet stuff, then including a small amount of dark chocolate in your diet can help with cravings while also having some health benefits. One Harvard study even found that having a small chunk of dark chocolate can help to lower blood pressure. Dark chocolate is also a source of antioxidants, as well as being good for the gut. It contains other minerals and vitamins, such as iron, magnesium, potassium, zinc, calcium, vitamin A and vitamin B. It does need to be good-quality dark chocolate with a high cocoa content – at least 60-70% or higher – and it should be consumed in small quantities, a couple of squares at a time, as it is still a source of saturated fat and sugar. But because it's less sweet than milk chocolate or white chocolate, it can be satisfying in much smaller amounts. You will need to look carefully at the ingredients label of any dark chocolate you're buying, as some varieties have added sugar or other additives to curb the bitter taste. Its main benefit, however, is that it gives you a sweet treat so that you don't feel like you're giving up everything you enjoy, and it's much better than eating large bars of highly processed milk chocolate.

OILY FISH

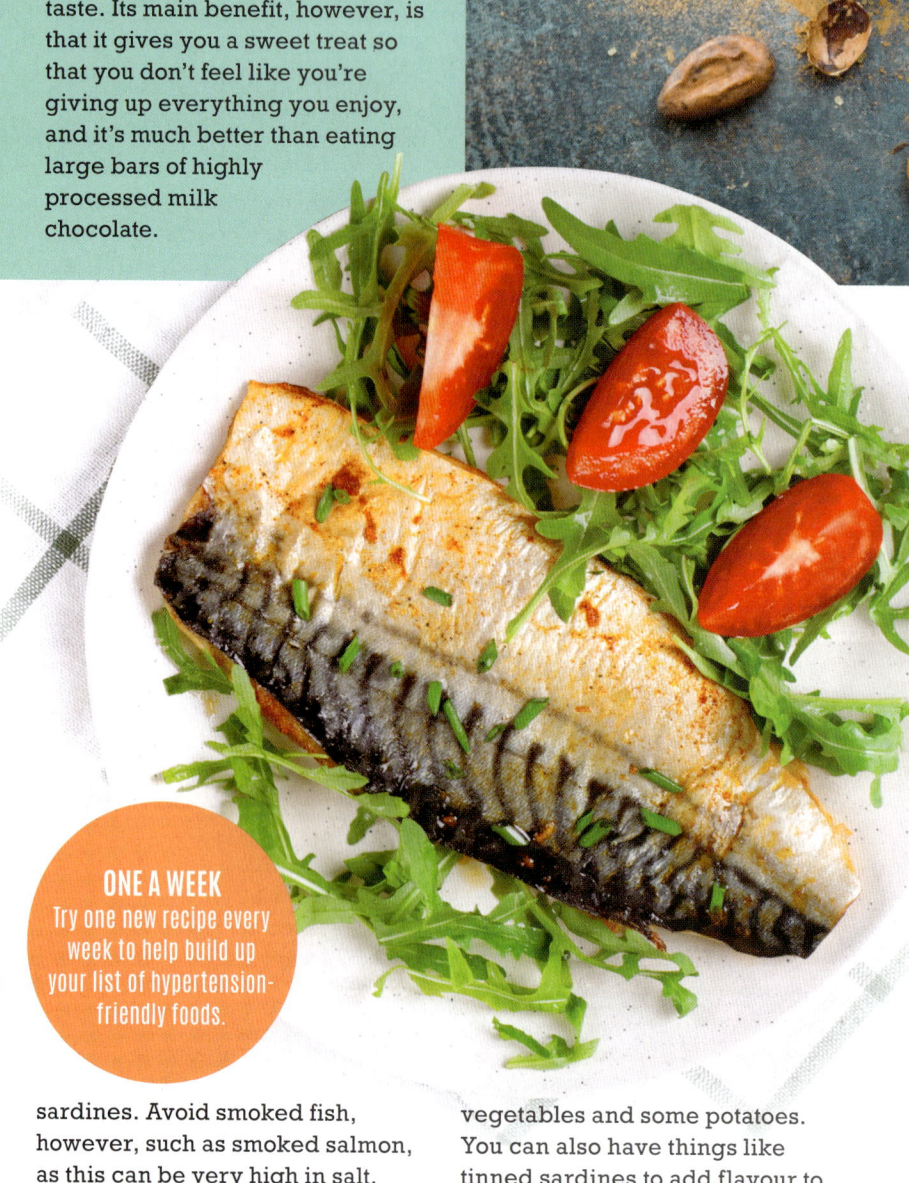

If you eat fish, it is a great addition to your diet when it comes to managing hypertension. It's recommended to eat at least two portions of fish a week, including one portion of oily fish. Oily fish is high in the polyunsaturated fat omega-3. Omega-3 has a huge number of health benefits, from brain health to eye function, and joint health to improvements in your skin. It's also really good for your heart health because it helps to lower triglyceride levels, improves your circulation and can help to prevent blood clots. It helps with lowering blood pressure and reducing your risk of cardiovascular disease, as well as being a source of vitamin D. Small fish where you also eat the bones, like whitebait or pilchards, are a great source of calcium. Oily fish includes things like salmon, mackerel, trout, herring and sardines. Avoid smoked fish, however, such as smoked salmon, as this can be very high in salt. Fresh fish is a great source of protein for your main meals, served simply with steamed vegetables and some potatoes. You can also have things like tinned sardines to add flavour to your salads. Fish can be baked too, which makes for a very simple and filling meal.

ONE A WEEK
Try one new recipe every week to help build up your list of hypertension-friendly foods.

104

TOP 10 FOODS FOR HYPERTENSION

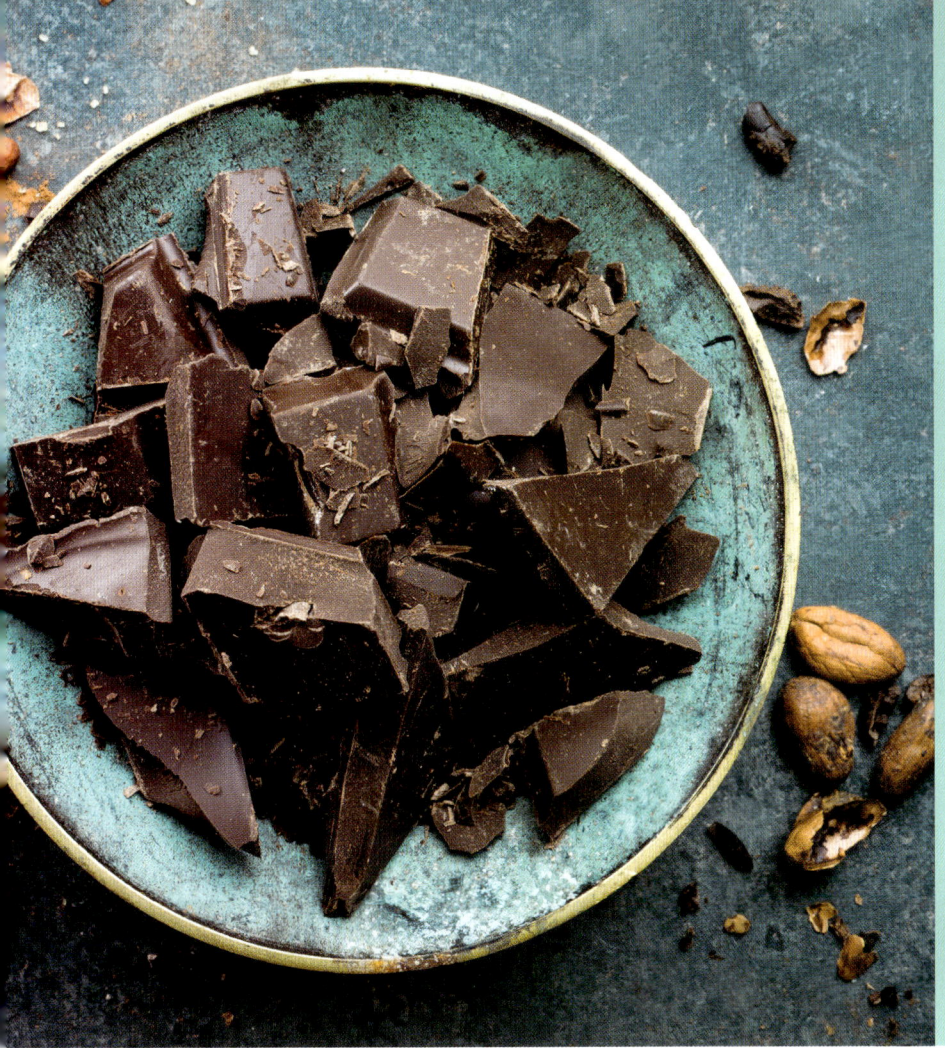

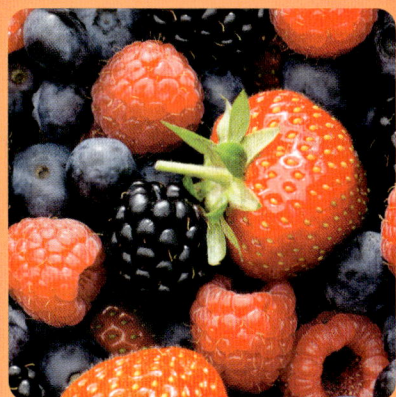

BERRIES

All fruits and vegetables are good to add into your diet when you're looking at lowering your blood pressure, but berries are particularly good. This is because they are full of nutrients, low in calories and very versatile. Berries are also good for fibre, vitamins and minerals. A study in the medical journal *Hypertension* (2021) with more than 900 participants found that eating about 1.6 servings of blueberries a day lowered systolic blood pressure. Berries are quite easy to incorporate into your diet. If you're having porridge for breakfast, then add a handful of berries on top. Eat them as a snack, either on their own or served with a low-fat Greek yoghurt. You can mix them into smoothies if you need a quick and easy on-the-go breakfast. Don't be afraid to use berries in savoury meals either. Strawberries and blueberries can be used to give a fresh edge to salads, and work especially well with spinach. Fresh berries can work out quite expensive, especially when they're not in season, so do look in the frozen section. You can buy packs of individual or mixed berries a lot cheaper, and they will keep for longer too. You could even grow your own in a garden or window box.

NUTS AND SEEDS

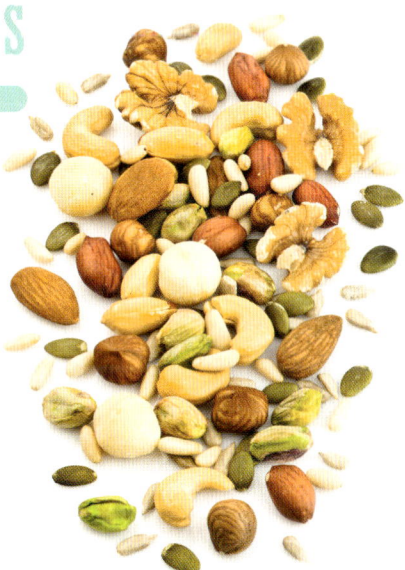

Nuts and seeds are a great addition to a healthy, balanced diet, though they are higher in calories, so you do need to be mindful about how many you're eating. Nuts and seeds are a great source of different minerals and nutrients, so eating a variety can give you the full range. It's even been shown that eating nuts and seeds can help to reduce cholesterol. Nuts and seeds are a great source of healthy fats. Seeds are good for sprinkling over yoghurt, porridge or salads, so consider adding things like pumpkin seeds, flaxseeds or sunflower seeds into your daily diet. They can help to boost your levels of magnesium, among other key minerals. When it comes to nuts, include things like walnuts, almonds and pistachios, which can all help with lowering blood pressure. They make a great snack on their own, but do make sure that you're only buying unsalted versions. You could even coat them in spices and roast them yourself to add some flavour and interest. You could make your own granola for a great breakfast option with a mixture of nuts and seeds, or use something like walnuts for a twist on the classic pesto (rather than pine nuts).

105

LIFESTYLE

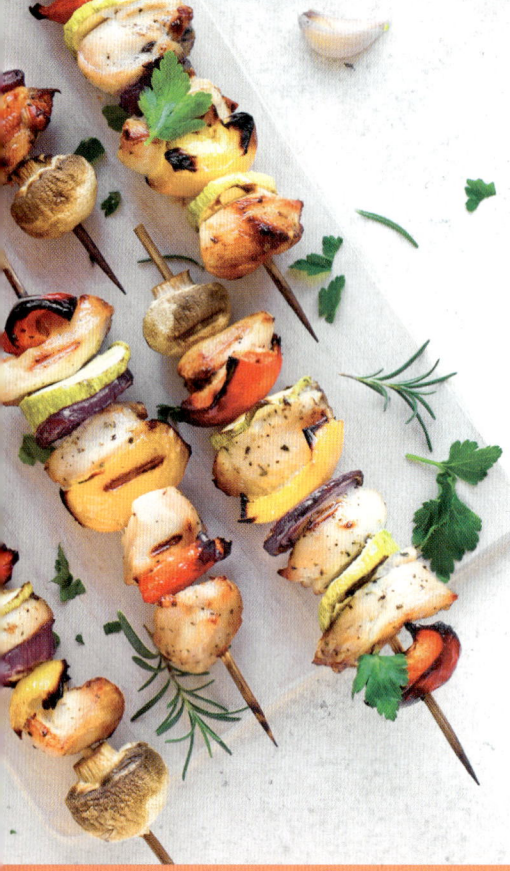

LEAN MEAT AND POULTRY

If you eat meat, then you should make sure you're eating lean options or opt for poultry. Both meat and poultry are great sources of protein, as well as being packed with essential micronutrients and vitamins. However, meat can be very high in saturated fat, which is why it's better to go for lean options. Red meat should be limited regardless, as this is linked to a greater risk of heart and circulatory diseases, as well as some cancers. If you enjoy red meat, choose the best quality cut that you can, trim any visible fat and cook without adding too much additional fat (like processed oils or butter). It can still have a place in a balanced diet. However, for everyday meals, lean pork or chicken is a better option, as these are perfect for those following the DASH or Mediterranean way of eating. Use your lean meat or poultry as the basis of your evening meal, and then add in a portion of wholegrain carbohydrates and plenty of colourful vegetables. You might also find it useful to roast a chicken, for example, at the weekend and slice it up to use in sandwiches or salads throughout the week – much better than processed ready-prepared meat products.

EAT THE RAINBOW
Try to eat a variety of different colourful fruits and vegetables every week.

OATS

Oats are simple, inexpensive and versatile, so they are a great option for anyone following a Mediterranean or DASH diet to help control blood pressure or lose weight. They are a source of soluble fibre, specifically beta-glucan, which can help to lower your cholesterol levels. They can also help to control your blood sugar and look after your gut health. Oats also contain a certain type of polyphenol that is both antioxidant and anti-inflammatory. It's thought that the polyphenols in oats can have a positive effect on blood pressure, according to data from one small study.[1] They are also very filling, which means that a portion of oats for breakfast could help you to reduce snacking in the morning and keep you satisfied for longer. You could top your porridge with other blood-pressure-friendly foods, like berries and a sprinkle of seeds. They're also good for making healthier flapjack or cereal bars at home, so you have something to grab in a hurry. You want to buy the least-processed oats you can. Instant oats, for example, have been milled to make them quick to cook, and sometimes they have added flavourings, salt or sugar. You are best going for rolled and steel-cut oats where possible, as these are the least processed.

TOP 10 FOODS FOR HYPERTENSION

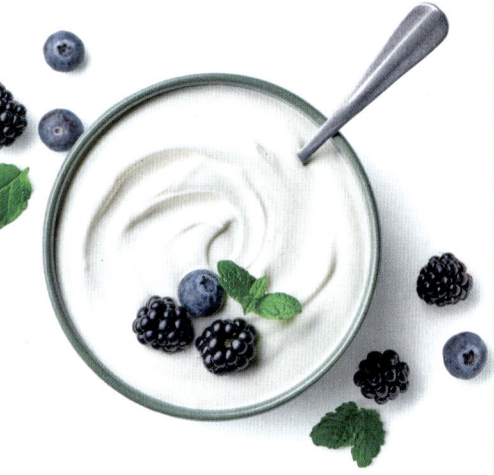

YOGHURT

Yoghurt is another food that should be in your fridge at all times. We're talking about natural, unsweetened and unflavoured yoghurt – the only ingredient should be milk. Yoghurt is made by heating milk and adding specific bacteria. This makes it really good for your gut health, and we know that looking after your gut helps with better health outcomes. There are lots of different types of yoghurt, but when it comes to managing hypertension, you want to look for one that's low fat or fat free. This means that you are getting the goodness of the calcium and protein, as well as the probiotics, but without the added calories and fat. Natural or Greek varieties are best. It can take time to get used to the flavour if you normally have sweetened yoghurt. You can use yoghurt to help thicken curries or stews; mix it with cucumber or mint to make a side sauce; use it as a swap for cream with desserts or simply with berries; or use it as a topping for porridge or cereal. You could even make your own, either with a yoghurt maker or on the hob. You only need milk and a 'starter', which is the live bacteria that ferments it (which, once you get going, can come from your last batch, or you can use a plain yoghurt with live cultures).

[1] Spencer J, et al. Chronic Vascular Effects of Oat Phenolic Acids and Avenanthramides in Pre- or Stage 1 Hypertensive Adults. Curr Dev Nutr. May 2020. **Images** Getty

5 FOODS TO AVOID

These foods are some of the worst culprits when it comes to impacting blood pressure

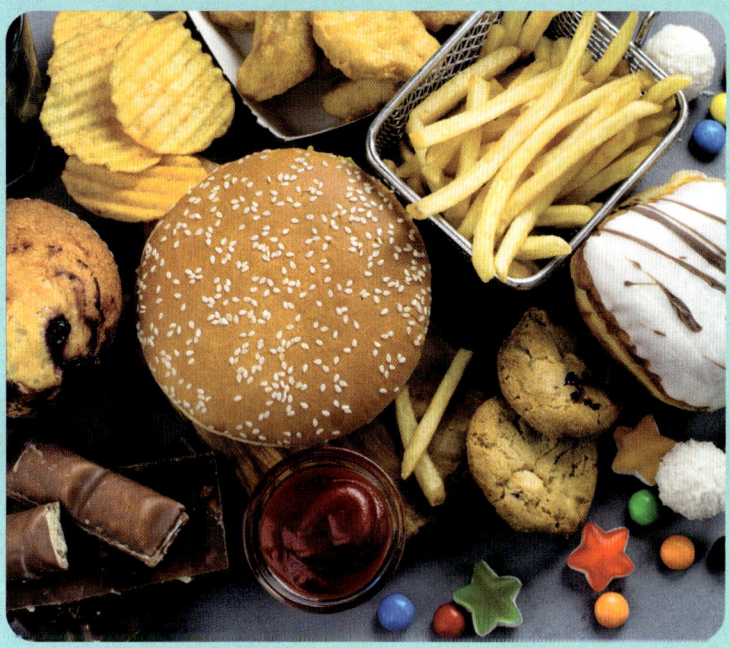

1. Processed meat
Processed meats are usually preserved using methods that result in high levels of salt. They can also be high in saturated fat. This includes things like sausages, bacon, sliced meats, burgers and hot dogs.

2. Sugary drinks
Sugary drinks give you a lot of calories without filling you up, so not only are you more likely to overconsume, you can easily go over your daily sugar allowance with just one drink.

3. White processed bread
Many of the breads that you get in the supermarket are highly refined, meaning that they are very high in salt. Where possible, switch to a wholegrain bread, buy it fresh or bake it yourself.

4. Table condiments
They might add flavour, but things like ketchup and salad dressing are adding salt to your meals, as well as extra calories. If you really can't give up your sauces, at least look for low-sodium versions.

5. Ultraprocessed snacks
Crisps, chocolate bars, sweets, cakes, biscuits… unfortunately these are all high in fat, sugar and salt, which means that they can contribute to high blood pressure. You can make your own healthier treats at home where you're in control of what goes in them.

RECIPES

Build the perfect plate for combatting high blood pressure, and get inspired by these great recipes

Now you know what you should be eating (and not eating), it's time to put it into practice and start building healthy meal plates that will support your health and help to reduce or manage your blood pressure.

Portion size and unbalanced plates are the two biggest issues that many of us face when it comes to dishing up our meals. If you're eating all the right foods but in the wrong portions, then you may find that you're consuming too many calories for your body. This means that while you will benefit from the goodness in your food, you could still be prone to weight gain, which is a risk factor for hypertension. And if your plate is made up of the wrong proportion of foods, you're not getting the optimum benefits from your diet.

The ideal healthy plate is made up of 50% fruits and vegetables. Ideally, as many of these as possible should be non-starchy vegetables, with a selection of different colours and textures. This helps to bulk out your meals and fill your plate, so that you feel like you're eating big portions. 'High volume and low calorie' is a great way to keep yourself satisfied and more likely to stay on track.

25% of your remaining plate should be for a source of protein, whether that's animal or plant based. So this is where you put a portion of lean meat, poultry, fish, tofu or lentils, for example. And the final 25% is for your carbohydrates, such as potato, brown rice or wholewheat pasta. You may then add a small amount of healthy fat or dairy.

Using this rough formula, you can build pretty much any meal you like! Even a simple sandwich can be created with bread (carbohydrate), a protein-based filling, a small amount of fat (avocado, butter, cheese) and a large side salad, served with a piece of fruit.

In this final section, we have selected a choice of recipes to get you started with your hypertension-friendly way of eating. We encourage you to give them a go and then, if you like, you can start to experiment – switch up the protein source, add a different carbohydrate, and mix up the herbs and spices…

Happy cooking!

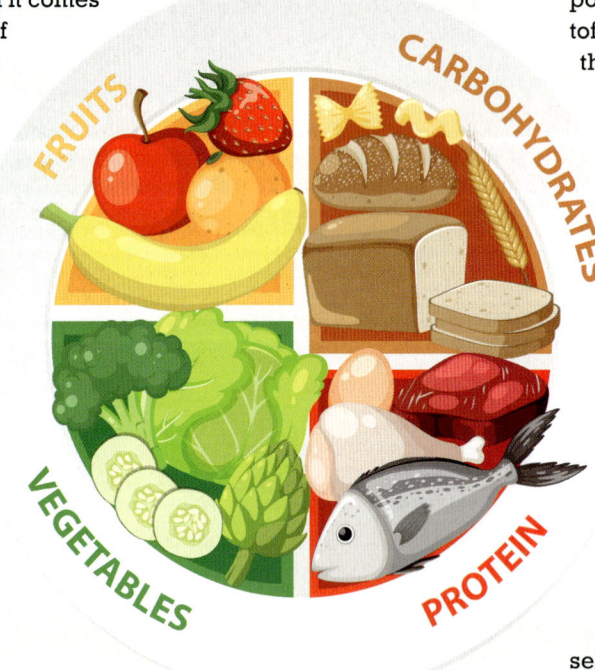

> "THE IDEAL HEALTHY PLATE IS MADE UP OF 50% FRUITS AND VEGETABLES"

110
CHOCOLATE AND HAZELNUT GRANOLA

112
SUPER BERRY BREAKFAST BOWL

114
SPICED CARROT AND LENTIL SOUP

116
TUNA AND LENTIL SALAD

118
SPICY BEEF AND LENTIL CHILLI

120
CHICKEN AND KALE STIR-FRY

122
SICILIAN-STYLE MACKEREL

124
OAT-AND-SESAME-CRUSTED SALMON WITH BLISTERED TOMATOES

126
VEGGIE CURRY WITH A MINTY YOGHURT

128
NUT, SEED AND BERRY CRUMBLE

SNAP YOUR FOOD
Take photos of meals you enjoy so you can build up a visual collection of food for when you're lacking inspiration.

RECIPES

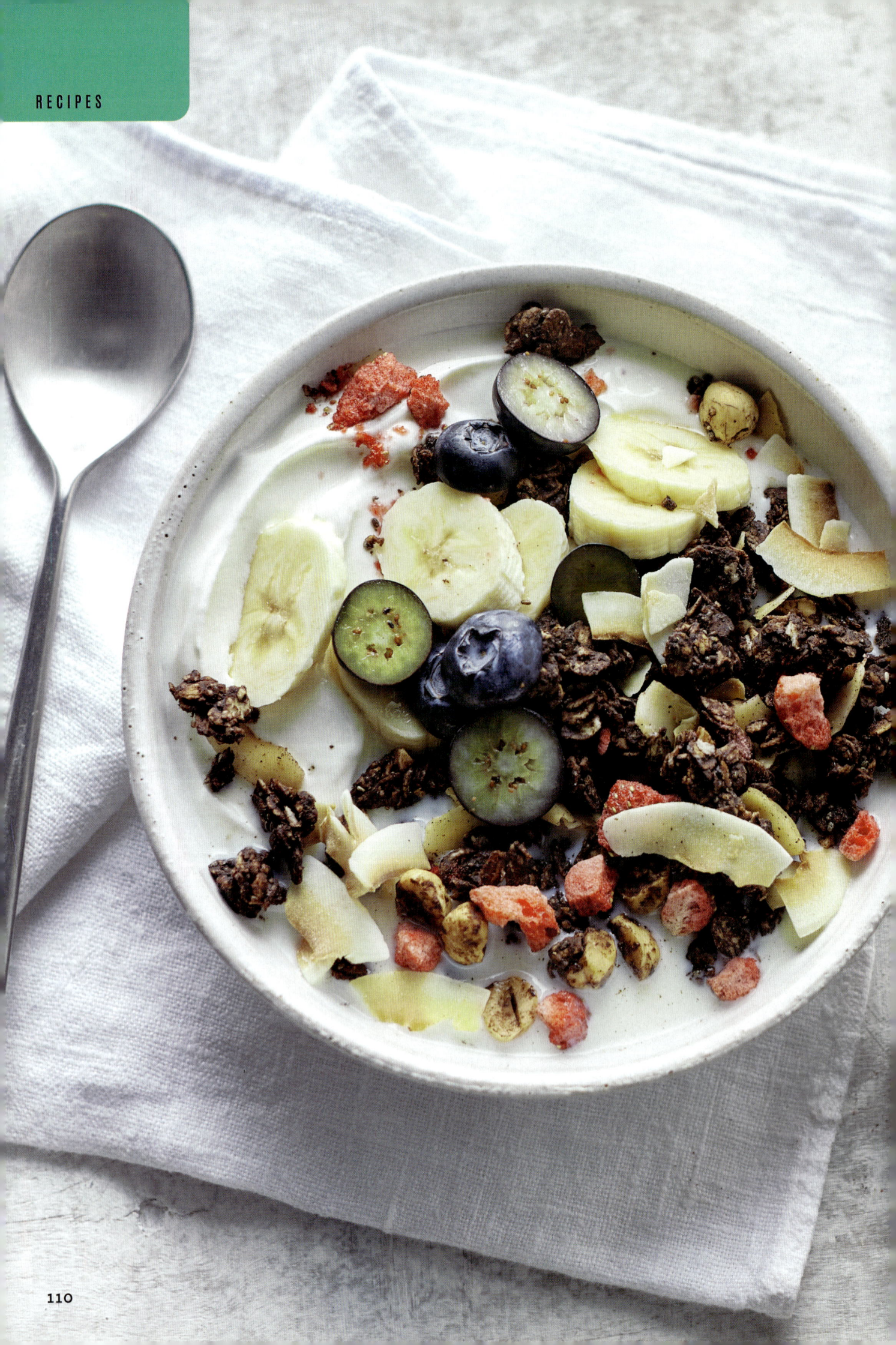

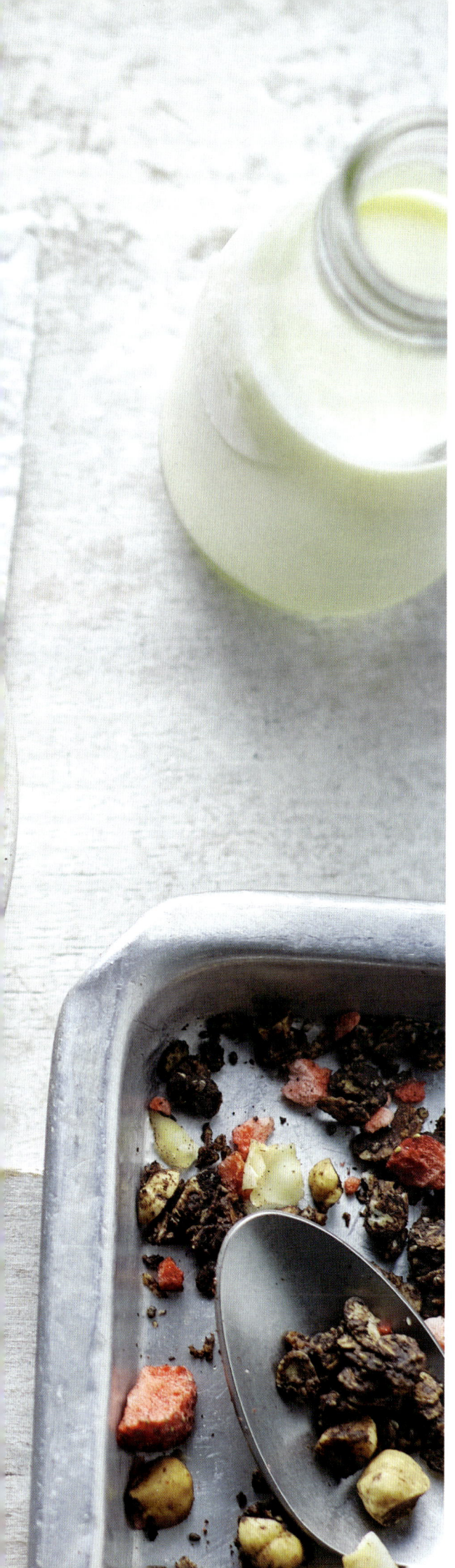

CHOCOLATE AND HAZELNUT GRANOLA

Mix and match this fibre-rich cereal to make it your own. Serve with fresh fruit and Greek yoghurt for extra protein

SERVES 6
READY IN 1 HR

200g (7oz) rolled oats
100g (3½oz) blanched hazelnuts, chopped
3tbsp cocoa powder
2tbsp mixed seeds (we used chia, sunflower and pumpkin)
2tbsp flaxseeds
2tsp ground cinnamon
5tbsp maple syrup
50g (2oz) coconut oil, melted
1tsp vanilla extract
1 egg white
50g (2oz) coconut flakes
3tbsp freeze-dried strawberries, lightly crushed (optional)
2tbsp cocoa nibs (optional)

1 Heat the oven to 180°C/350°F/Gas 4. In a large bowl, mix the oats, chopped hazelnuts, cocoa powder, seeds, and cinnamon.
2 In a jug, whisk together the maple syrup, coconut oil and vanilla extract. Add to the dry ingredients and mix everything together.
3 Next, whisk the egg white until white and frothy, then fold into the granola. This makes the granola extra crunchy, but you can leave it out if you prefer.
4 Spread the mixture in an even layer on a lined baking tray and bake for 25 mins. Toss in the coconut flakes and bake for another 10-15 mins until crisp and golden. Leave to cool on the tray.
5 Break the granola into small clusters, and add the strawberries and cocoa nibs, if using.

Baking granola in batches is cheaper and healthier than buying it. The granola can be stored in an airtight container for two to three weeks.

Shop-bought granola contains more added sugar, salt and excess fats, so it is healthier to make your own if you can.

RECIPES

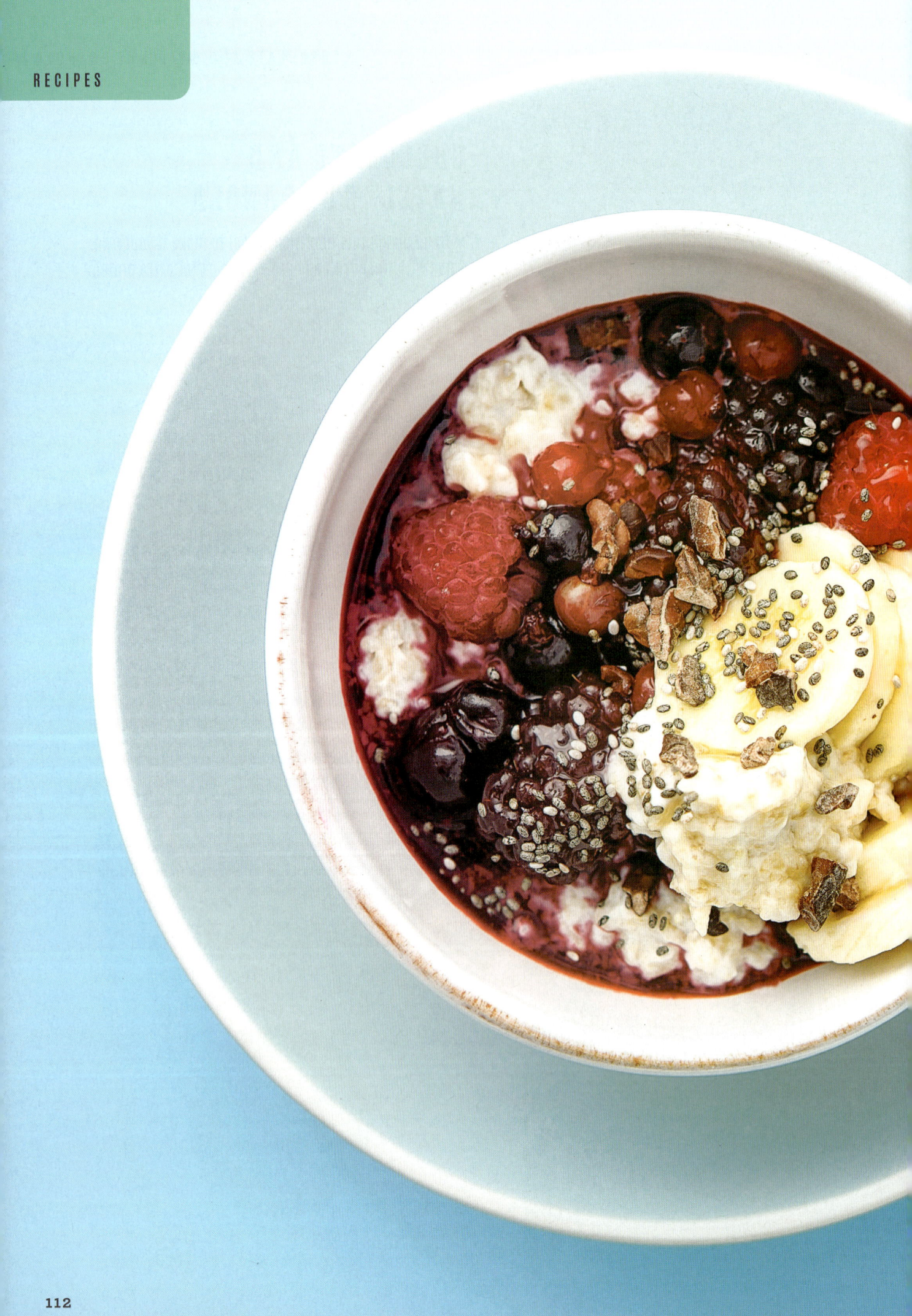

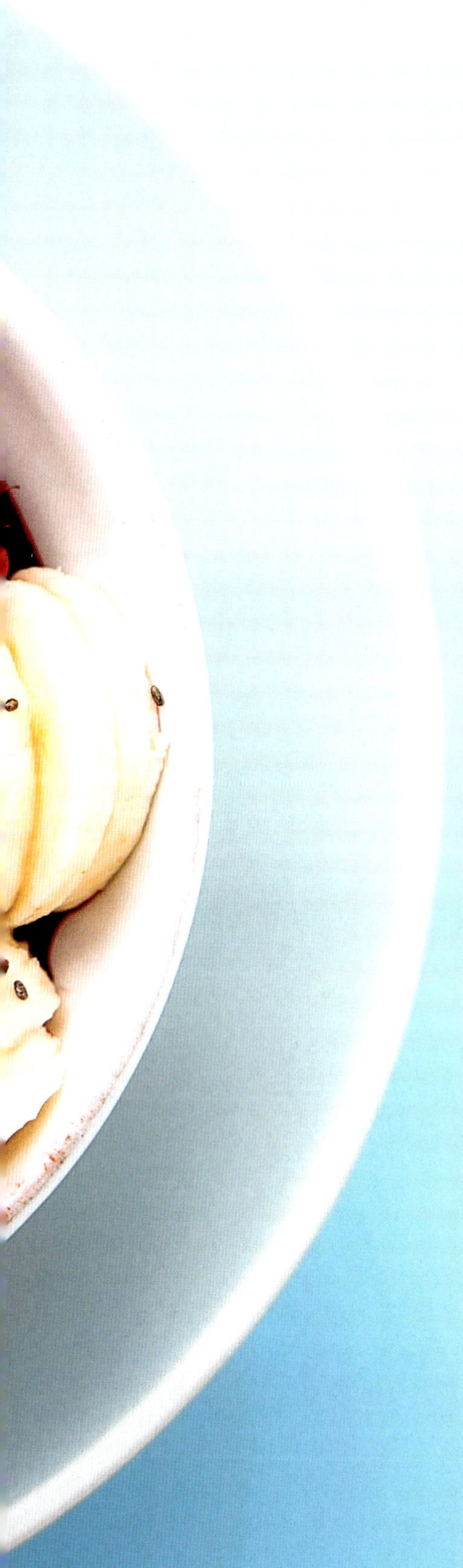

SUPER BERRY BREAKFAST BOWL

The chia seeds and walnuts here add a lovely textural contrast to the oats and compote

SERVES 6
READY IN 25 MINS

80g (3oz) frozen berries
Zest ½ orange and a squeeze of juice
50g (2oz) oats
100ml (3½fl oz) Greek yoghurt

¼ banana, sliced
½tsp chia seeds
½tsp coca nibs
25g (1oz) walnuts, chopped
Handful berries to garnish

1 Put the frozen berries, orange zest and juice into a small pan and cook on a medium heat for 5 mins until the berries have softened.
2 Stir the oats into the yoghurt and leave to sit for 15 mins. Top with the warm berries and garnish with banana, chia seeds, cocoa nibs, walnuts and some extra berries.

Chia seeds are not only rich in omega-3 fatty acids, but they are also an easy way to get more beneficial dietary fibre - just 2-3tbsp will provide nearly 10g fibre.

RECIPES

SPICED CARROT AND LENTIL SOUP

This flavourful soup is packed with vitamins A and K, as well as fibre

SERVES 2
READY IN 35 MINS

300g (10½oz) carrots, scrubbed and chopped
60g (2½oz) red split lentils
750ml (1½pt) hot vegetable stock
½tsp ground coriander
2tbsp soured cream
¼tsp coriander seeds, crushed

1 Put the carrots in a pan with the lentils, stock and ground coriander, and season with ground black pepper. Bring to the boil and simmer for 25 mins until the carrots are tender.
2 Pour the soup contents into a blender and whizz until it's smooth.
3 Pour the soup into a bowl and add a spoonful of soured cream in the centre. Top with a sprinkling of crushed coriander seeds.

> Red lentils are a great plant-based protein full of nutrients such as folate and potassium. Add them to soups for a filling, low-fat meal.

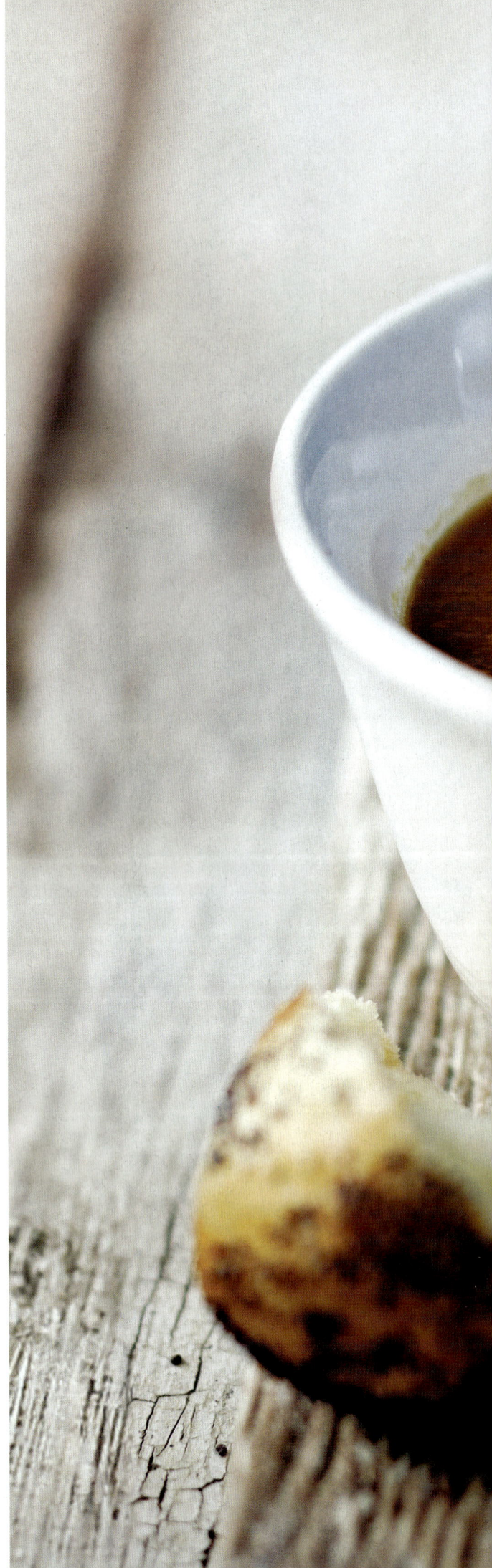

SPICED CARROT AND LENTIL SOUP

RECIPES

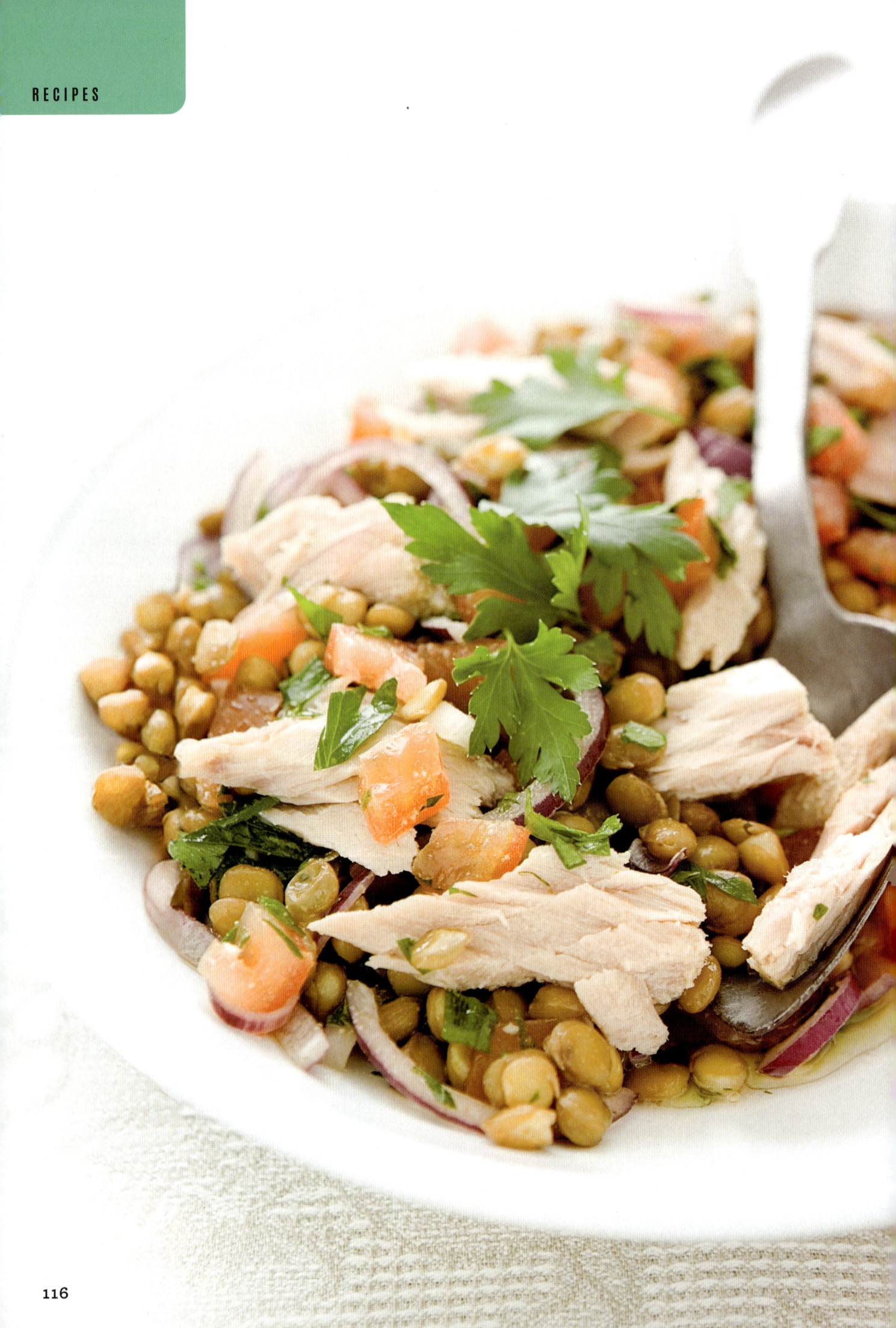

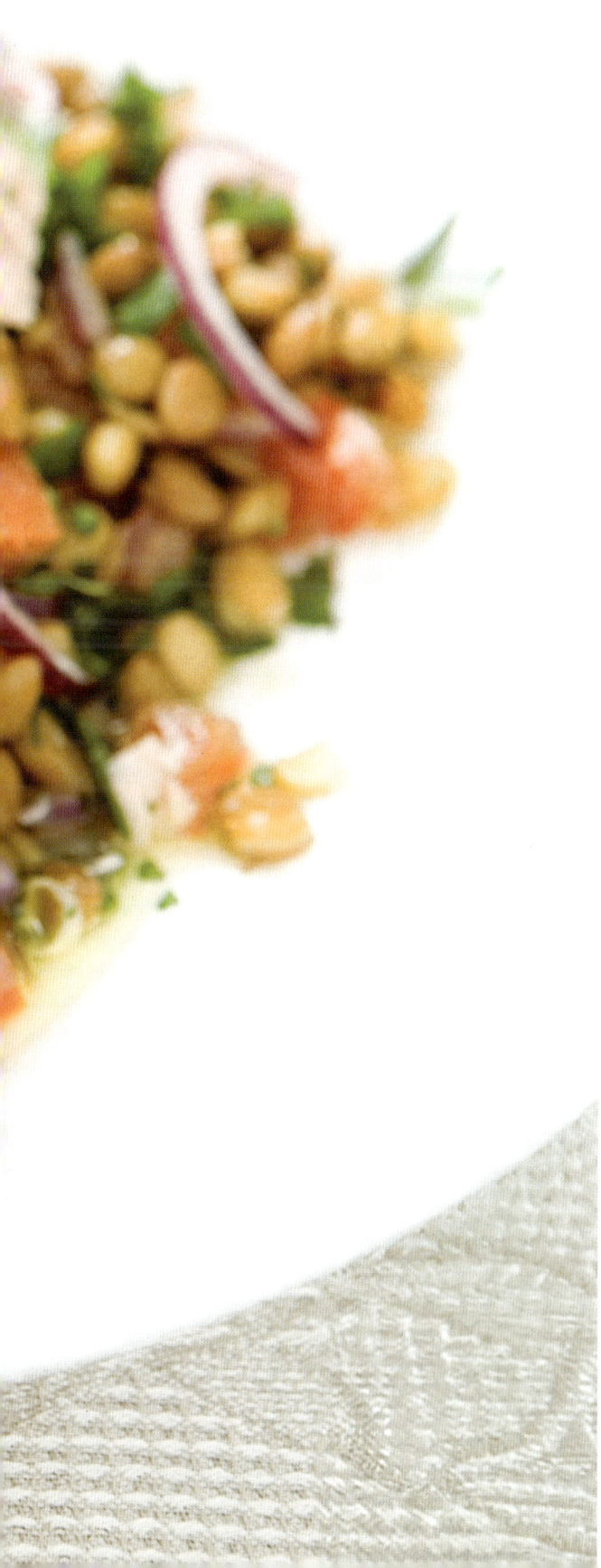

TUNA AND LENTIL SALAD

A heart-healthy lunch that's high in protein and fibre

SERVES 4
READY IN 10 MINS, PLUS INFUSING

200g (7oz) jar or tin tuna in olive oil
3tbsp olive oil
2tbsp lemon or lime juice
1 small red onion, peeled and finely sliced
1 garlic clove, peeled and crushed
½tsp ground cumin or cumin seeds, toasted
400g (14oz) tin lentils, rinsed and drained
2 plum tomatoes, rinsed and finely chopped
4tbsp chopped flat-leaf parsley
Crusty bread, to serve

1 Whisk 2tbsp oil from the tuna with the olive oil and lemon juice in a large bowl. Add the onion, garlic and cumin and then the lentils. Leave for 30 mins if you have time to allow the flavours to infuse.
2 Stir in the chopped tomato, flaked tuna and parsley, and season with freshly ground black pepper. Serve with crusty bread.

Although not considered an oily fish, tinned tuna is a high-quality and inexpensive source of protein, and contains many vitamins and minerals.

RECIPES

SPICY BEEF AND LENTIL CHILLI

Opt for lean beef mince and add lentils for healthy comfort food

SERVES 4
READY IN 1 HR

500g (1lb) lean beef mince
1tbsp olive oil
1 onion, finely chopped
1 stick celery, finely chopped
1tsp each ground coriander, paprika, cayenne pepper and oregano
100g (3½oz) red lentils
400g (14oz) tin chopped tomatoes
1 beef stock cube, dissolved in 600ml (20fl oz) water
400g (14oz) tin kidney beans, rinsed and drained
Rice, to serve
Soured cream, coriander and lime wedges to garnish

1 Dry-fry the mince in a non-stick pan. Set aside. Add the oil to the pan and fry the onion and celery for 10 mins.
2 Return the mince to the pan and add the spices and oregano. Stir for 1 min, then add the lentils, tomatoes and stock.
3 Simmer for 45 mins, adding the beans for the last 15 mins. Serve chilli with rice. Garnish with soured cream and coriander, with lime wedges on the side.

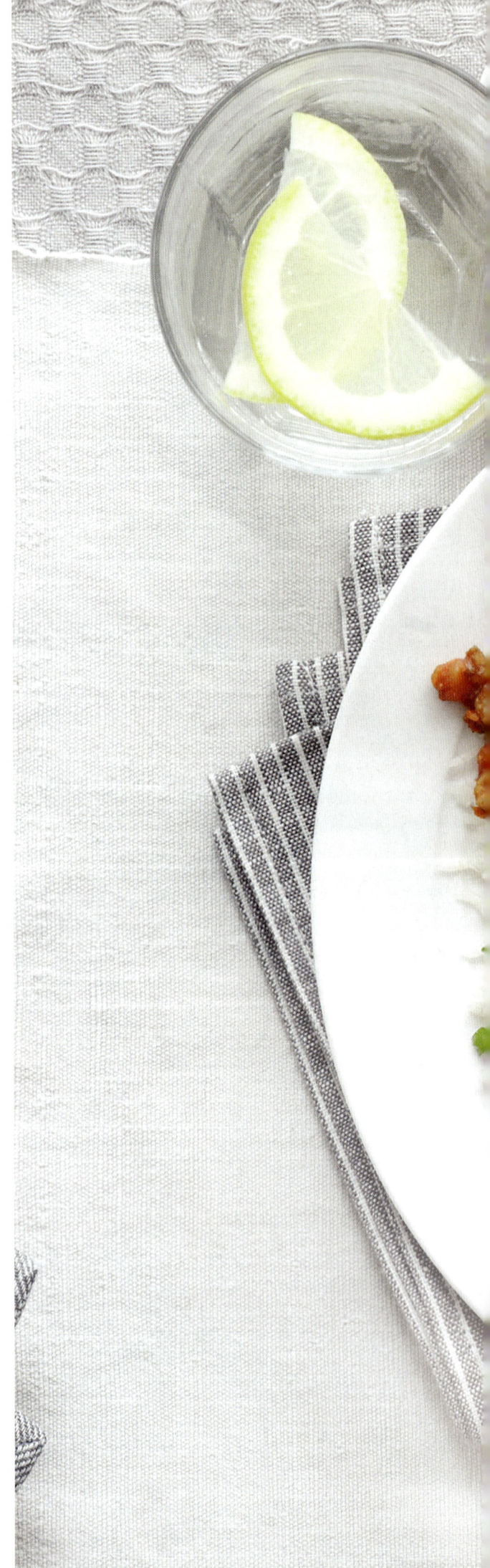

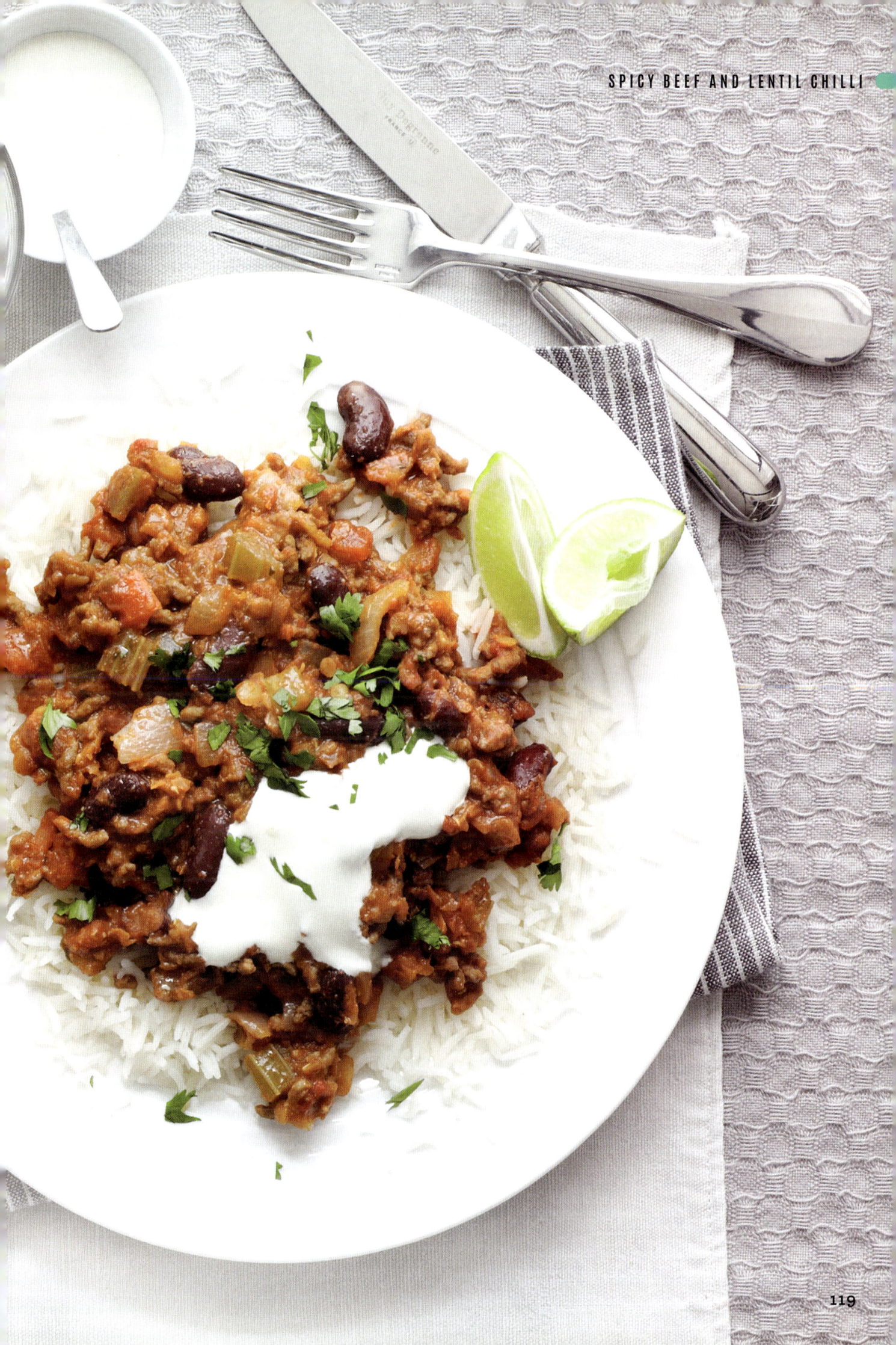

SPICY BEEF AND LENTIL CHILLI

RECIPES

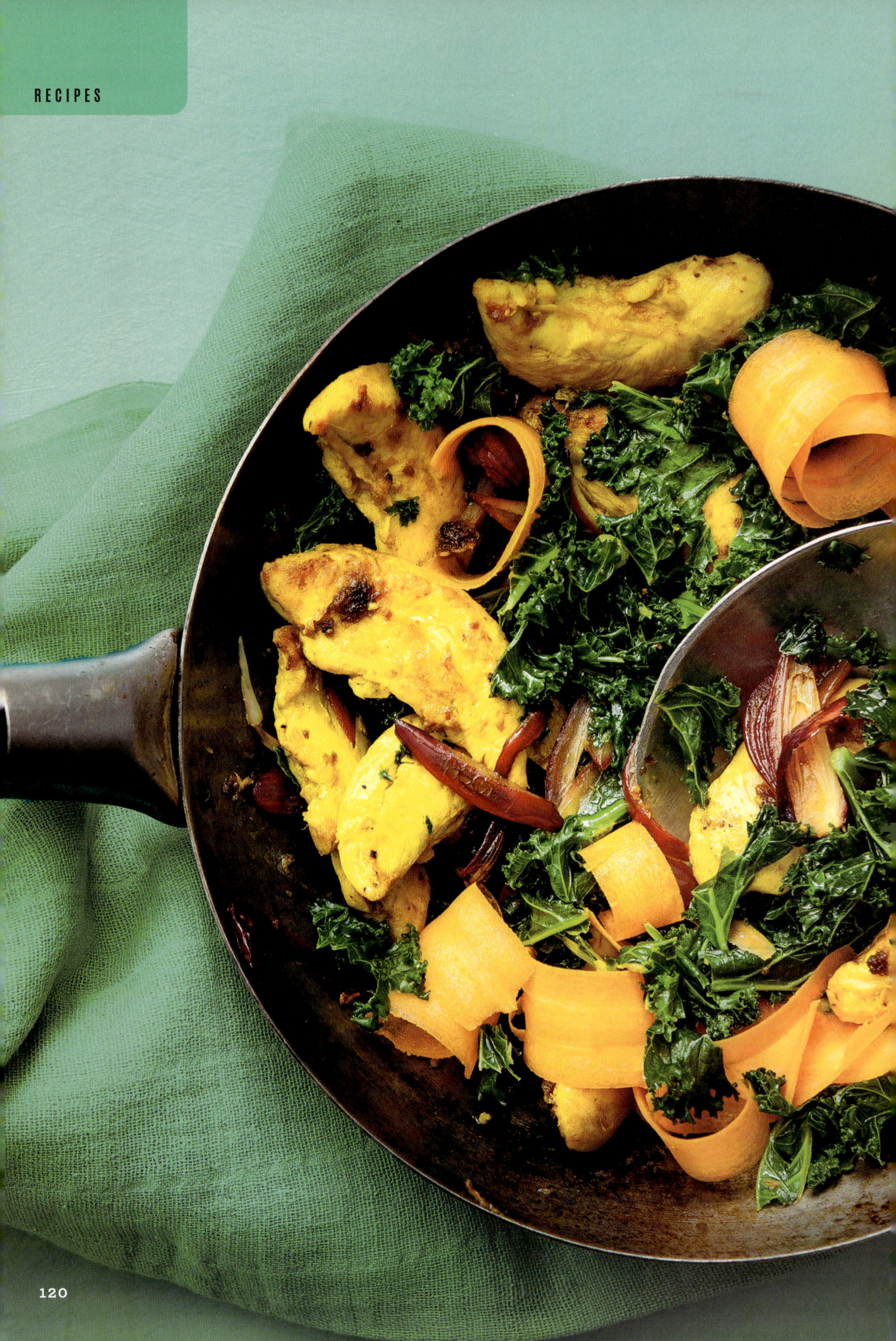

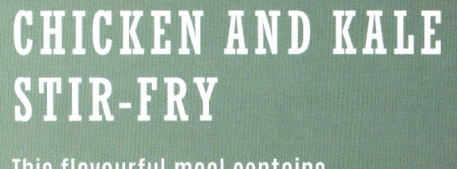

CHICKEN AND KALE STIR-FRY

This flavourful meal contains anti-inflammatory turmeric and miso

SERVES 6
READY IN 1 HR

425g (15oz) pack mini chicken breast fillets
2½cm (1in) fresh ginger, grated
2 garlic cloves, peeled and grated
Finely grated zest and juice of 1 lemon
2tbsp rapeseed oil
¼tsp turmeric
2 red onions, sliced
250g (9oz) chopped curly kale
2tbsp miso paste
2 carrots, cut into ribbons with a vegetable peeler

1 Put the chicken in a shallow dish. Add the ginger, garlic, lemon zest and juice and stir well to mix. Leave to marinate for 30 mins.
2 Heat the oil in a wok or large frying pan, add the chicken and cook for 3 mins to brown. Sprinkle over the turmeric, stir well and cook for a further 3 mins.
3 Push the chicken to one side and add the sliced onions. Cook for 3 mins to soften slightly.
4 Add the kale. Stir the miso paste into 200ml (7fl oz) boiling water and pour over the kale, cover and cook for 3 mins. Add the carrots and cook for 2 mins more before serving.

Stir-fries are a great way to bulk up your meals with plenty of veg and protein. Plus they feel like a healthy takeaway!

RECIPES

SICILIAN-STYLE MACKEREL

A delicious recipe of light and clean-tasting fresh mackerel

SERVES 4
READY IN 25 MINS

5tbsp extra virgin olive oil
4 large or 8 small, very fresh mackerel fillets
1 small red onion, halved and finely sliced
200g (7oz) cherry tomatoes
1 garlic clove, sliced
3tbsp red wine vinegar
2½tbsp caster sugar
1 heaped tbsp capers, rinsed and drained
2tbsp golden raisins or sultanas
2tbsp pine nuts, toasted
Handful of flat-leaf parsley leaves
Crusty bread, to serve

1 Put 2tbsp of the olive oil in a large frying pan set over a medium-high heat. Add the mackerel fillets, skin-side down, and sear for 2 mins, until the skin is golden and crisp.
2 Carefully turn over the fish, cook for 1-2 mins, depending on size, then remove to a plate and set aside. Turn the heat down a little, add the onion and cook, stirring often, for 5 mins.
3 Stir in the tomatoes and garlic, and cook for a further 2 mins. Add the red wine vinegar, sugar, capers, raisins and pine nuts and simmer for 1 min or so. Season to taste, then return the fish to the pan.
4 Warm through, then drizzle with the remaining olive oil and scatter the parsley over. Serve with the crusty bread.

Oily fish like mackerel contains omega-3 fatty acids, which can help to lower your blood pressure.

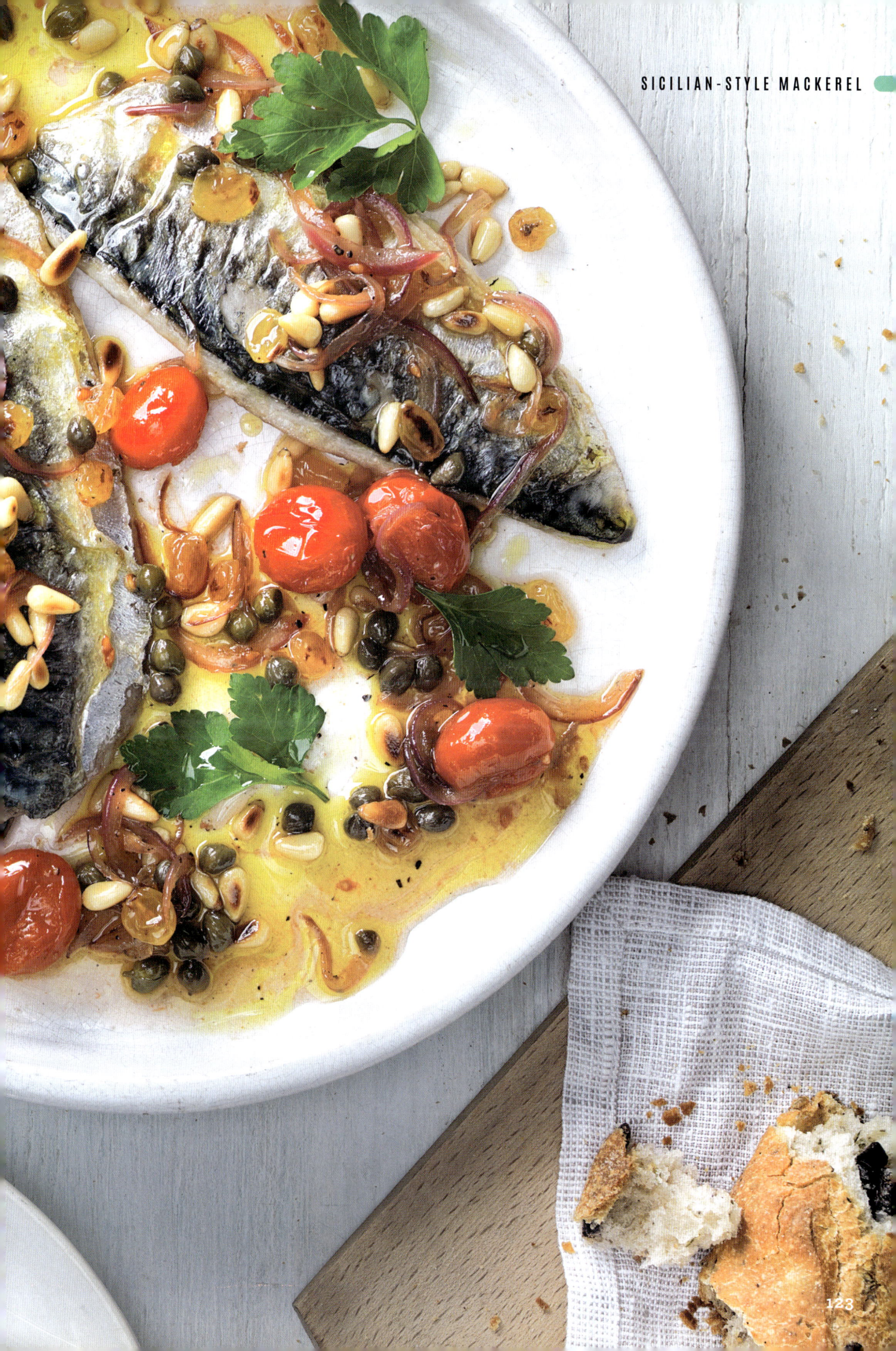

SICILIAN-STYLE MACKEREL

RECIPES

OAT-AND-SESAME-CRUSTED SALMON WITH BLISTERED TOMATOES

The salmon and seeds are a tasty way to get omega-3, which is shown to help lower blood pressure

SERVES 4
READY IN 30 MINS

4tbsp oatmeal
1tsp oregano, chopped, or ¼tsp dried oregano
4tbsp sesame seeds
1½ lemons
4 skinless salmon fillets (about 140g (5oz) each)

2tbsp olive oil
2 courgettes, trimmed and cut into sticks
1 garlic clove, crushed
200g (7oz) cherry tomatoes on the vine

1 Heat the oven to 180°C/355°F/Gas 4. Combine the oatmeal, oregano and sesame seeds in a shallow dish. Squeeze the juice of 1 lemon into another shallow dish.
2 Dip the fish in the lemon juice then the oatmeal mixture, turning to coat, then arrange on a lined baking tray and drizzle with 1tbsp of the olive oil. Bake for 15 mins, until golden.
3 Toss the courgettes with the garlic and the remaining oil. Spread over another baking tray. Roast for 15 mins.
4 Cut the remaining half lemon into wedges and add to the fish tray, along with the tomatoes. Turn the courgettes and return both trays to the oven for another 10 mins.

Flaxseeds, nuts, seeds and seaweed are sources of omega-3 for vegetarians and vegans, so swap the salmon here for a protein of your choice.

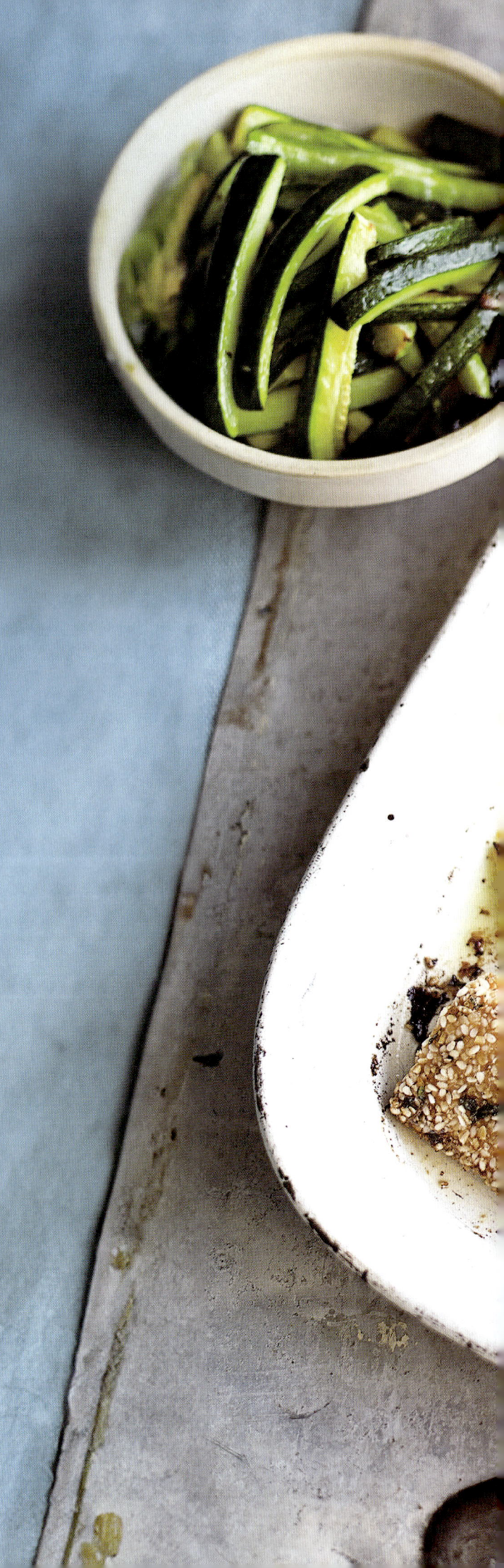

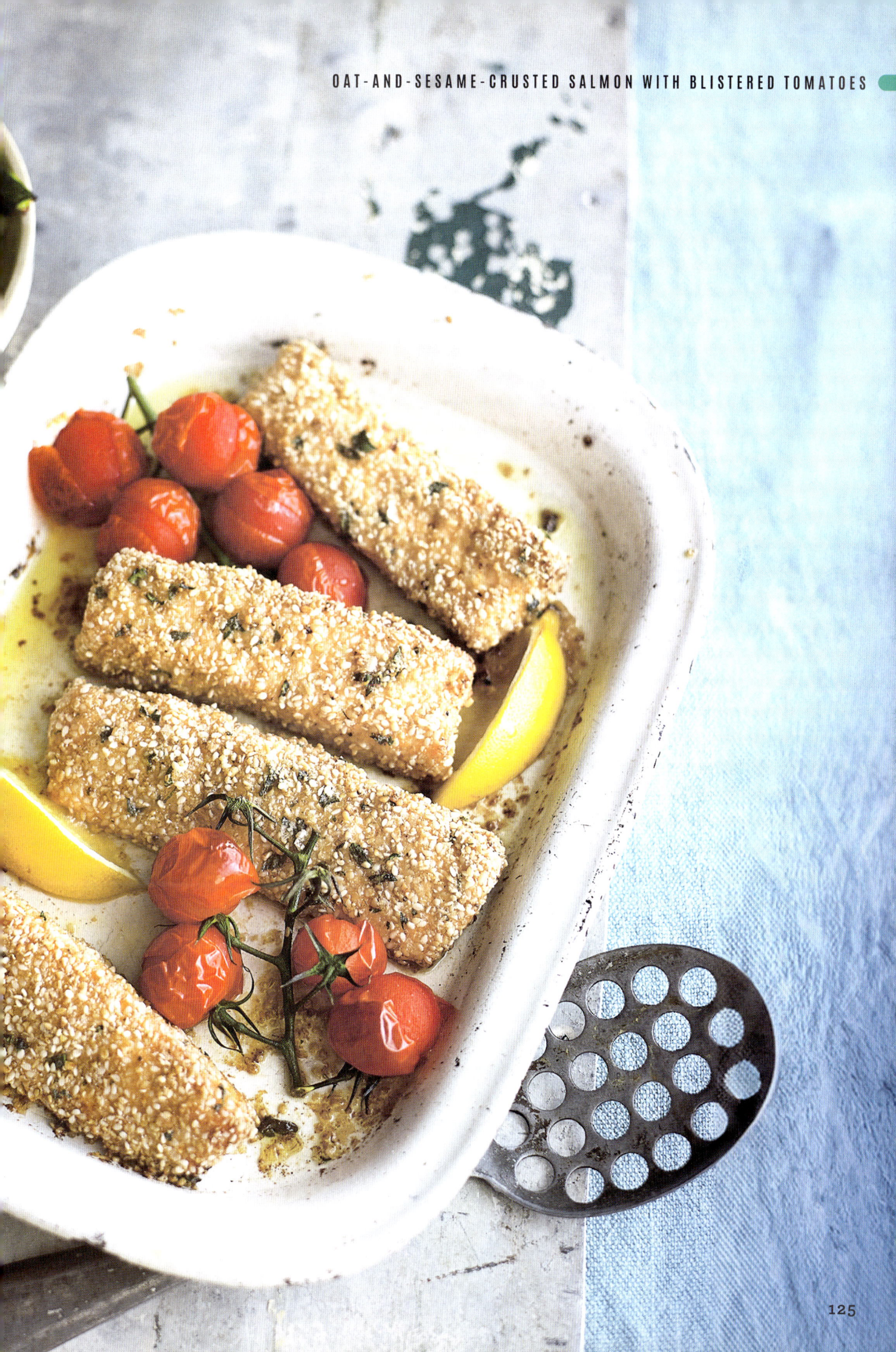

OAT-AND-SESAME-CRUSTED SALMON WITH BLISTERED TOMATOES

RECIPES

VEGGIE CURRY WITH A MINTY YOGHURT

Our fully loaded vegetable curry takes a little while to prepare but is well worth the effort

SERVES 4
READY IN 1 HR 10 MINS

½ butternut squash, peeled, seeds removed, and cut into **3cm (1¼in)** pieces
1 aubergine, cut into chunks
3tbsp rapeseed oil
1 small onion, diced
1 carrot, peeled and diced
200g (7oz) passata
400ml (14fl oz) tin coconut milk
½ cauliflower, cut into florets
150g (5oz) Brussels sprouts, trimmed and quartered
1 red chilli, deseeded and diced

2 large naan bread, or 4 small ones
2tbsp toasted, flaked almonds
120g (4oz) natural yoghurt mixed with **1tbsp** chopped fresh mint

FOR THE PASTE
½tbsp coriander seeds
½tsp cumin seeds
4 cloves
1tsp dried chilli flakes, or more if you like it hot
1 star anise
½tsp ground turmeric
1tbsp ground ginger

½tbsp coconut sugar
3 garlic cloves, crushed
1tbsp apple cider vinegar

FOR THE CRISPY KALE
4 leaves curly kale, roughly chopped
6 small dried curry leaves
½tsp black mustard seeds
1tbsp olive oil

1 For the paste, dry-fry the coriander seeds, cumin seeds, cloves, chilli flakes and star anise until intensely aromatic. Grind to a fine powder in a pestle and mortar. Add the turmeric, ginger, coconut sugar and garlic. Pummel to crush the garlic, then add the vinegar and mix to make a paste.
2 Toss the squash and aubergine in 2tbsp oil, season and fry in batches until browned on all sides.
3 Heat the remaining 1tbsp oil in a separate large pan, add the onion and carrot, and cook gently until softened. Stir in the passata and simmer for 10 mins until thickened.
4 Stir the curry paste into the pan then gradually stir in the coconut milk. Fill half the tin with water and add this too. Bring to the boil and then reduce to a simmer.
5 Mix in the cauliflower, Brussels sprouts and chilli, cover and simmer for 10 mins. Add the squash and aubergine, and cook for a further 20 mins, until the vegetables are tender.
6 Meanwhile, heat the oven to 220°C/425°F/Gas 7. Place the kale in an ovenproof dish with the curry leaves and mustard seeds, and drizzle over the oil. About 10 mins before the curry is ready, cook the kale in the oven until crisp.
7 Heat the naan bread in the oven for 2 mins. Stir the flaked almonds into the curry. Serve the curry with the kale crumbled on top, and the mint yoghurt and naan bread on the side.

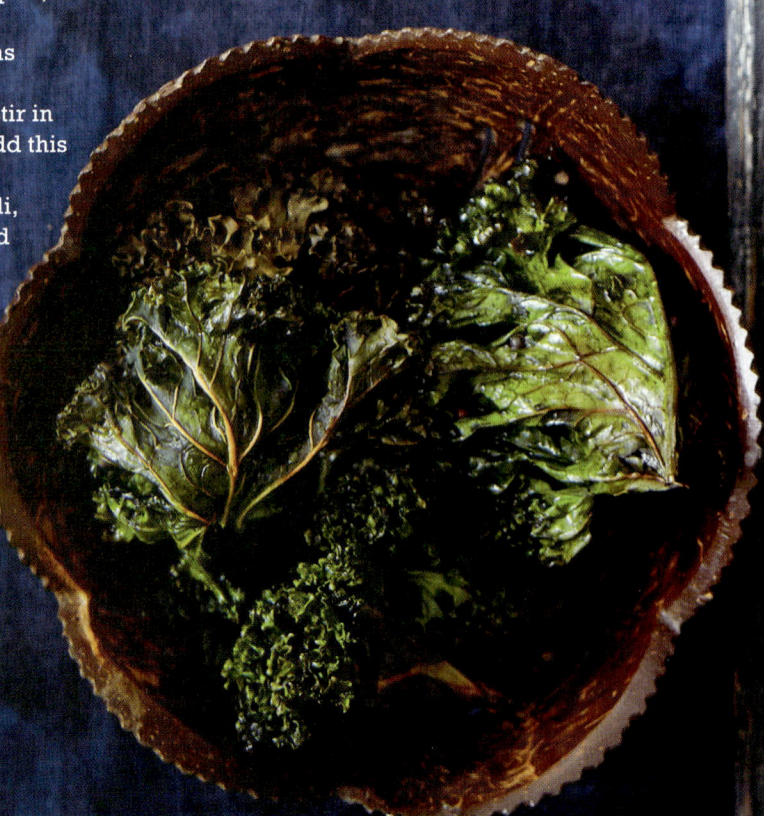

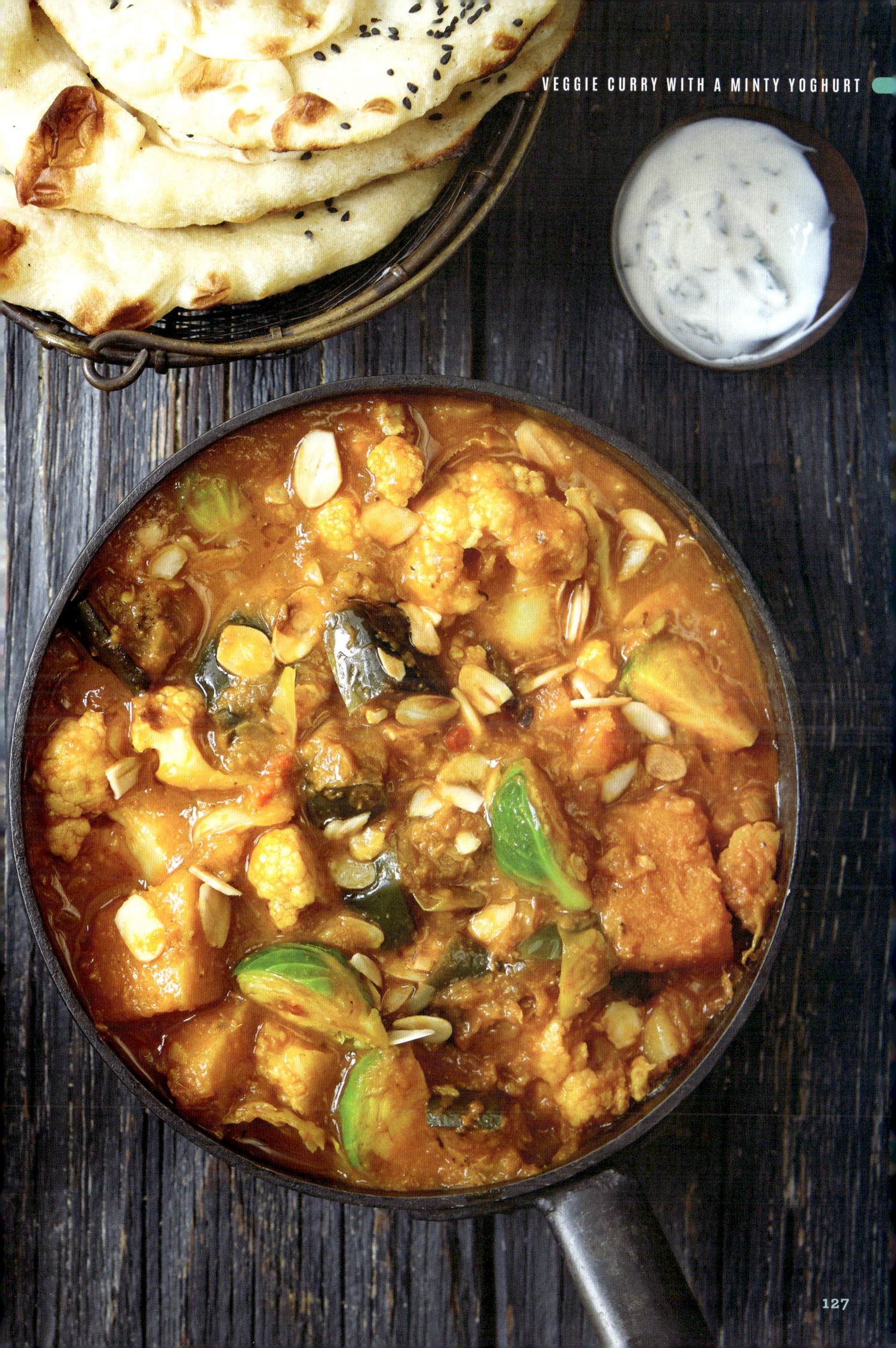

VEGGIE CURRY WITH A MINTY YOGHURT

RECIPES

NUT, SEED AND BERRY CRUMBLE

Add texture and flavour to an old favourite, with the addition of nutritious nuts and seeds

SERVES 6
READY IN 55 MINS

6 apples, peeled and cut into chunks
4tbsp maple syrup
250g (9oz) blueberries

FOR THE TOPPING
80g (3oz) butter
100g (3½oz) quinoa flakes
50g (2oz) rolled oats
4tbsp light brown sugar
50g (2oz) nuts
1tsp ground cinnamon
2tbsp each sesame, sunflower and pumpkin seeds
Half-fat crème fraîche, to serve

1 Heat the oven to 200°C/400°F/Gas 6. Toss the apples in the maple syrup on a baking tray and bake for 15 mins.
2 Meanwhile, make the topping. Rub the butter into the quinoa flakes and oats until it resembles coarse breadcrumbs. Stir in the sugar, nuts, cinnamon and seeds.
3 Put the apples in an ovenproof dish and stir in the blueberries, then top with the crumble topping. Return to the oven and bake for 25 mins.
4 Once the crumble is golden and bubbling, remove and serve with crème fraîche.

Blueberries are packed with anthocyanins, which are thought to help reduce blood pressure.

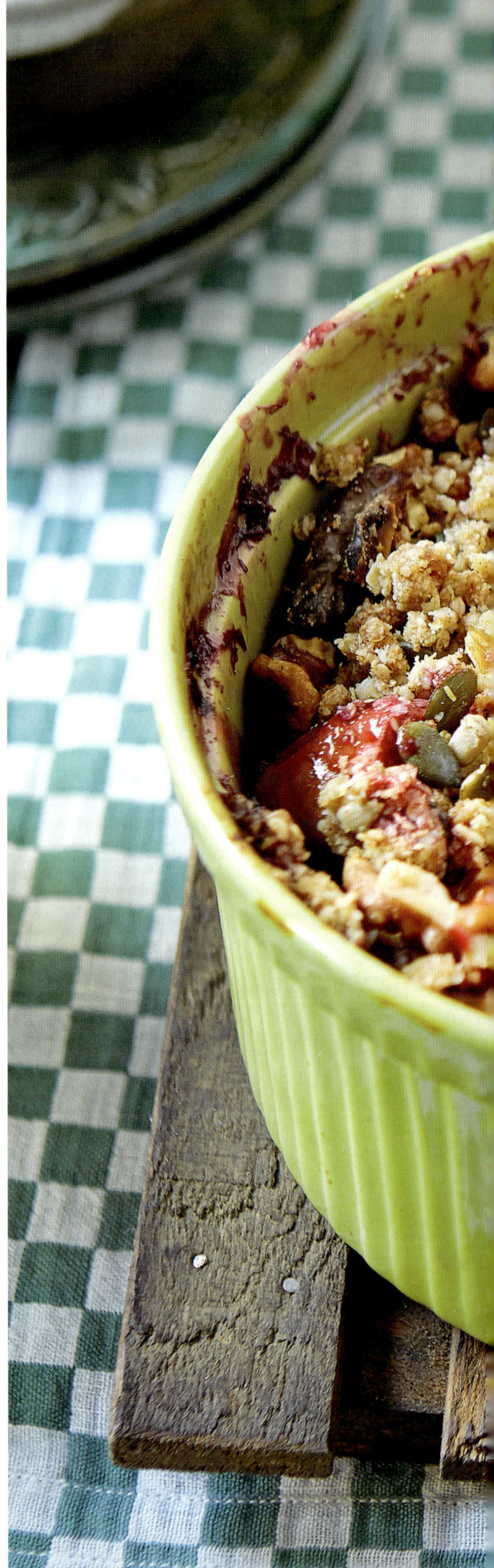

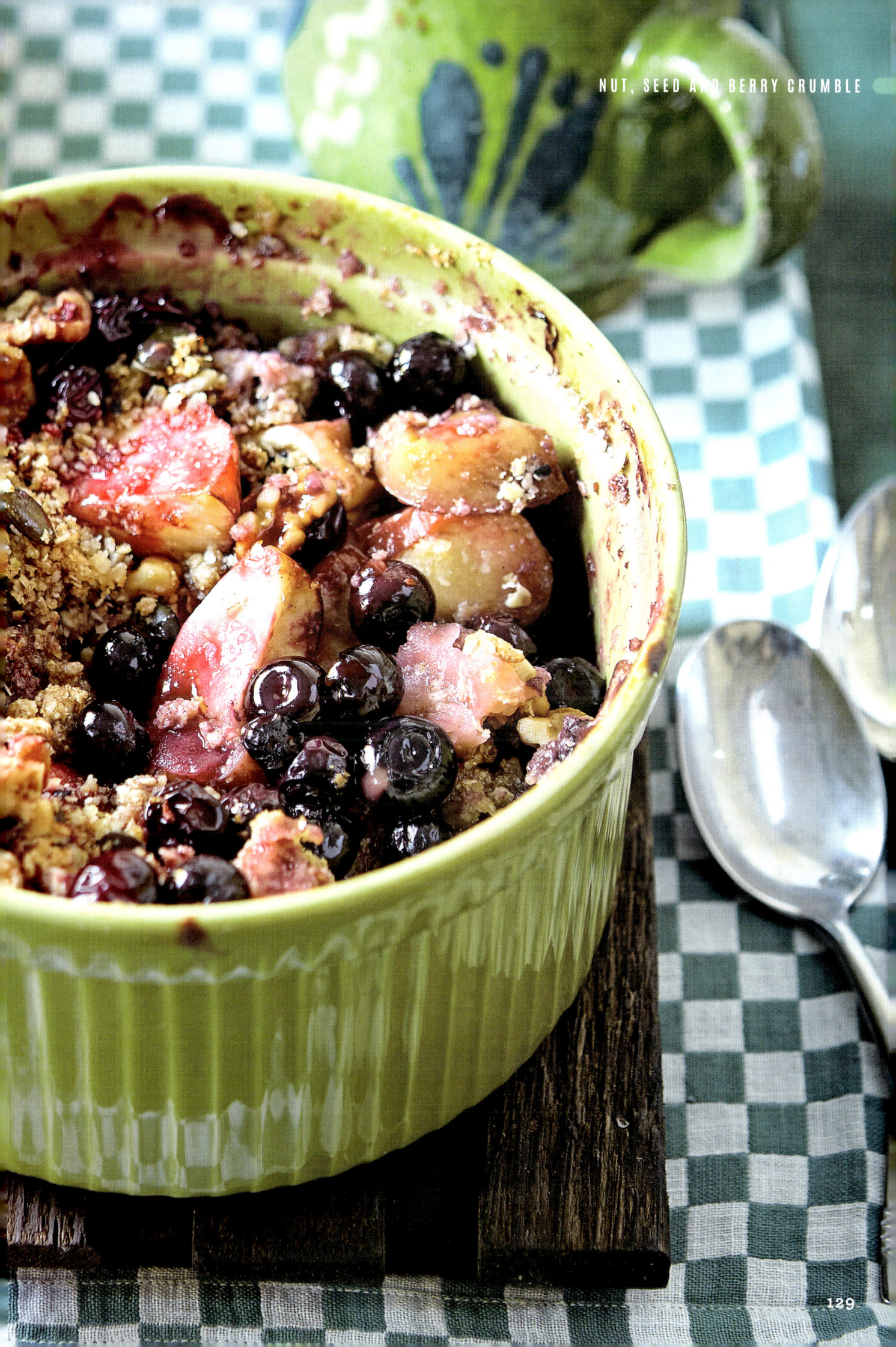

NUT, SEED AND BERRY CRUMBLE

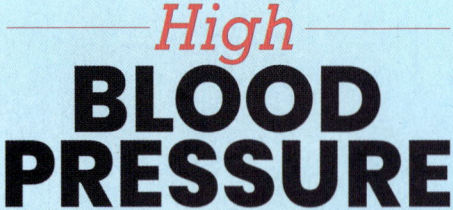

High BLOOD PRESSURE HANDBOOK

Future PLC Quay House, The Ambury, Bath, BA1 1UA

Editorial
Author **Julie Bassett**
Group Editor **Sarah Bankes**
Art Editor **Lora Barnes**
Head of Art & Design **Greg Whitaker**
Editorial Director **Jon White**
Managing Director **Grainne McKenna**

Contributors
Jo Cole, Andy Downes, Adam Markiewicz, Dan Peel

Cover images
Getty Images

Photography
All copyrights and trademarks are recognised and respected

Advertising
Media packs are available on request
Commercial Director **Clare Dove**

International
Head of Print Licensing **Rachel Shaw**
licensing@futurenet.com
www.futurecontenthub.com

Circulation
Head of Newstrade **Tim Mathers**

Production
Head of Production **Mark Constance**
Production Project Manager **Matthew Eglinton**
Advertising Production Manager **Joanne Crosby**
Digital Editions Controller **Jason Hudson**
Production Managers **Keely Miller, Nola Cokely, Vivienne Calvert, Fran Twentyman**

Printed in the UK

Distributed by Marketforce – www.marketforce.co.uk
For enquiries, please email: mfcommunications@futurenet.com

Disclaimer
This publication is for information only and is not intended to substitute professional medical advice and should not be relied on as health or personal advice. Never disregard professional advice or delay seeking it.

Always consult your pharmacist or doctor for guidance and before using any natural, over-the-counter or prescription remedies, and read any instructions carefully.

In an emergency, call the emergency services and seek professional help immediately.

Readers rely on any information at their sole risk, and High Blood Pressure Handbook, and its publisher, Future Publishing Ltd, limit their liability to the fullest extent permitted by law.

High Blood Pressure Handbook First Edition (LBZ6980)
© 2024 Future Publishing Limited

We are committed to only using magazine paper which is derived from responsibly managed, certified forestry and chlorine-free manufacture. The paper in this bookazine was sourced and produced from sustainable managed forests, conforming to strict environmental and socioeconomic standards.

All contents © 2024 Future Publishing Limited or published under licence. All rights reserved. No part of this magazine may be used, stored, transmitted or reproduced in any way without the prior written permission of the publisher. Future Publishing Limited (company number 2008885) is registered in England and Wales. Registered office: Quay House, The Ambury, Bath BA1 1UA. All information contained in this publication is for information only and is, as far as we are aware, correct at the time of going to press. Future cannot accept any responsibility for errors or inaccuracies in such information. You are advised to contact manufacturers and retailers directly with regard to the price of products/services referred to in this publication. Apps and websites mentioned in this publication are not under our control. We are not responsible for their contents or any other changes or updates to them. This magazine is fully independent and not affiliated in any way with the companies mentioned herein.

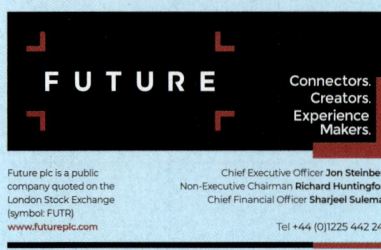

Future plc is a public company quoted on the London Stock Exchange (symbol: FUTR)
www.futureplc.com

Chief Executive Officer **Jon Steinberg**
Non-Executive Chairman **Richard Huntingford**
Chief Financial Officer **Sharjeel Suleman**

Tel +44 (0)1225 442 244

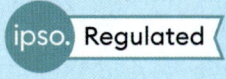